PRAISE FOR. . .
How Hope, Love, and
In A Maze Called Alzheimer's

"A moving account of one man's journey from a conventional faith to a stunningly real relationship with God, this spiritual memoir will linger in your imagination long after you have finished reading it. It describes the author's path through the desert of his beloved wife's slow descent into Alzheimer's disease for more than sixteen years. *A Path Revealed* is an intimate meditation on how one man was shown how to love and trust God in the midst of devastating loss."

—DEBORAH VAN DEUSEN HUNSINGER, PhD, Charlotte W. Newcombe Professor of Pastoral Theology at Princeton Theological Seminary. Her most recent book, *Bearing the Unbearable: Trauma, Gospel and Pastoral Care*, was awarded the 2015 Book of the Year by the Academy of Parish Clergy.

———————

"Carlen Maddux and his wife, Martha, visited with me for a week's retreat shortly after she was diagnosed with Alzheimer's disease. The story Carlen tells is an amazing journey. It would require that Carlen be willing to risk, to set aside the blocks of disbelief and distrust, to open his mind and heart to possibilities he'd never have imagined.

"Carlen is a good, clear writer. His choice of words is precise, his images effective. Everything about this story rings true, authentic, intimate, and experiential."

—SR. ELAINE M. PREVALLET, SL, retreat director with the Sisters of Loretto in Kentucky. She is the author of three books, including *Making the Shift: Seeing Faith Through a New Lens*.

———————

"This book is a solid core of hope within a tale of seeming woe. Almost everyone knows someone who suffers from Alzheimer's, or who loves someone who suffers from Alzheimer's. Carlen Maddux spent seventeen years in that chronic crucible of one step forward, three steps back.

He's come through it—and without letting his true love go. How was this possible? Carlen's odyssey is a trip that one man has made. Yet without knowing it, he has made it for us all. It's an emotional journey, a geographical journey, a medical journey, and a spiritual journey."

—THE REV. DR. PAUL F.M. ZAHL, Episcopal minister, is author or co-author of ten books, including *Grace in Practice* and *PZ's Panopticon*, and producer of the popular *PZ's Podcasts* at http://www.mbird.com/tag/pzs-podcast/.

"At age 50, Martha Maddux was visited by the surprising, upending presence of one of life's most dreaded diseases. Surely we—all of us—would dread facing and embarking on a similar heart-wrenching wilderness pilgrimage. But should we have to, our broken places will be made stronger along the precarious way, through the compassionate and vulnerable witness of Martha and her family's ministry to us, and its compelling honesty and spiritual depth which urge us to walk with thanksgiving 'into the deep we call God.'"

—REV. DR. DEAN K. THOMPSON, President and Professor of Ministry Emeritus, Louisville Presbyterian Theological Seminary

---

"Scripture tells us that hope does not disappoint because of the love of God. Carlen Maddux's compelling book, *A Path Revealed*, reaches out beyond crisis to the unbounded hope, love, and joy of the Lord. It does not disappoint. Maddux's fine work connects the dots of a spiritual journey, and inspires us to reach higher."

—GREG O'BRIEN, diagnosed with early onset Alzheimer's, describes his experience in his riveting, first-person account *On Pluto: Inside the Mind of Alzheimer's*. His book has won the 2015 Beverly Hills International Book Award for Medicine, the 2015 International Book Award for *Psychology Today's* "Health," and is an Eric Hoffer International Book Award finalist.

"The reader who travels with Carlen into the mysterious depths of human life, human tragedy, and human relationships will be led to reflect, to ponder, and to expand. Carlen is a strong writer. He invites us to share—to share his journey, to share his discovery of how his search led his mind and soul beyond problem-solving into acceptance, peace, celebration, and gratitude."

—REV. DR. ARTHUR ROSS III, pastor emeritus of White Memorial Presbyterian Church in Raleigh, North Carolina, and former chair of the board of trustees at Union Presbyterian Seminary.

A PATH REVEALED

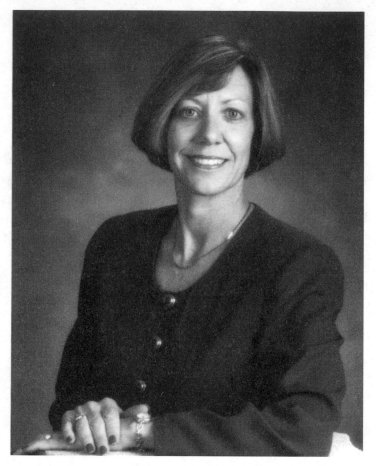

Martha Cooper Maddux

CARLEN MADDUX

A PATH
REVEALED

HOW HOPE, LOVE, AND JOY

FOUND US

DEEP IN A MAZE

CALLED **ALZHEIMER'S**

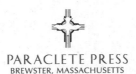

PARACLETE PRESS
BREWSTER, MASSACHUSETTS

2016 First printing

A Path Revealed: How Hope, Love, and Joy Found Us Deep in a Maze Called Alzheimer's

Copyright © 2016 by Maddux Report L.C.

ISBN 978-1-61261-784-8

Unless otherwise indicated, biblical quotations are from the Revised Standard Version, Second Edition, 1971 copyright by the National Council of the Churches of Christ of the United States of America, Division of Christian Education, and published in The New Oxford Annotated Expanded Edition, 1977.

Biblical quotations marked KJV are taken from the Authorized King James Version of the Holy Bible.

The Paraclete Press name and logo (dove on cross) are trademarks of Paraclete Press, Inc.

The photograph of Martha Cooper Maddux found on page iv was taken by Lisa Munafo, D & L Photography.

Library of Congress Cataloging-in-Publication Data

Names: Maddux, Carlen, author.
Title: A path revealed : how hope, love, and joy found us deep in a maze
    called Alzheimer's / by Carlen Maddux.
Description: Brewster MA : Paraclete Press Inc., 2016.
Identifiers: LCCN 2016022327 | ISBN 9781612617848 (trade paper)
Subjects: LCSH: Alzheimer's disease--Religious aspects--Christianity. |
    Alzheimer's disease--Patients--Religious life. | Alzheimer's
    disease--Patients--Care. | Maddux, Martha Cooper, -2014. | Maddux, Carlen.
Classification: LCC BV4910.6.A55 M33 2016 | DDC 248.8/6196831--dc23
LC record available at https://lccn.loc.gov/2016022327

10 9 8 7 6 5 4 3 2 1

Published by Paraclete Press
Brewster, Massachusetts
www.paracletepress.com

Printed in the United States of America

To our children,
David, Rachel, and Kathryn,
and their families

For Martha and her legacy

In appreciation of my family,
my late parents, Margaret and Dave,
my late sister, Alice, and
my brother, Bob, and his family

CONTENTS

Part Three

THE WAY OF INTIMACY 99

FOREWORD

A foreword is sort of a blessing or stamp of approval to assure prospective readers that the author offers a voice worth hearing. That is why Carlen Maddux invited me, as a longtime friend, a former pastor to him and his family, and a discussion partner as this book emerged, to accept this assignment. I gladly agreed. Carlen and his family have been treasured friends since the mid-1980s, a friendship that has persisted for twenty years beyond the time I left his community and moved to another state.

The Carlen I know and respect is the "real thing"—a solid person of inquiring faith for all of his adult life, a former college athlete, an intelligent and respected businessman and community leader, and a father, husband, and friend. Over a seventeen-year period, I witnessed Carlen in a new role: caregiver to an incurably ill wife, Martha, whom he loved deeply and with whom he enjoyed life. That role confronted Carlen with his limitations, his failings, and his accumulated pain. Such confrontations are often inescapable in this life. When they occur, some people grow up; others grow down. In this book, Carlen tells a memorable story of growing up. I have followed the story with great sadness and great admiration, from its very beginning.

The theme of Carlen's story is captured by a small piece of needlepoint another friend made for me forty-plus years ago. Mounted in an oval frame, with a small owl in the lower corner, the sampler reads, "Life is a mystery to be lived, not a problem to be solved."

Carlen tells of his wife's tragic journey through Alzheimer's. Soon after learning of the diagnosis, Carlen began an intense effort to solve the problem created by the disease. Could it be treated in any way? When the search for that answer reached a dead end, he was faced with another question: how could he understand this tragedy, making sense out of a senseless event? That journey also proved impossible. As Carlen's story unfolds, readers are led away from problem-solving into mystery and into discovering the power that embracing mystery can bring to this human experience.

Carlen's journey not only takes us to monasteries, hospital rooms, and Australia, but also leads us into the dark depths of family dysfunction, a reality in Carlen's and Martha's lives. The journey creates new relationships between Carlen and his children, and with Martha and her parents. The journey leads into Carlen's soul; we join him in discovering the ways a life of faith includes radically new understandings of that treasured, sacred word.

The reader who travels with Carlen into the mysterious depths of human life, human tragedy, and human relationships will be led to reflect, to ponder, and to expand. Carlen is a strong writer.

One of his strengths is that, as he tells this story, his words invite us into conversation. His style invites dialogue between reader and author. Carlen does not seek to convince others of anything, certainly not anything that could be called "religious." Rather, he invites us to share—to share his journey and his discovery of how his search led his mind and soul beyond problem-solving into acceptance, peace, celebration, and gratitude.

As you read this book, reflect on the difference between being smart and being wise. When Carlen began the journey, people who knew him would quickly classify him as being smart. When the book concludes, Carlen is wiser, and his readers have been given the opportunity to grow in wisdom as well. Wisdom is a spiritual attribute, one that emerges through experience, reflection, dialogue, debate, revelation, and resolution—not resolution as in solving a math problem, but resolution as it occurs in poetry, music, or prayer.

My one-word response to this book is gratitude—gratitude for Martha's life, gratitude for Carlen's love toward Martha, gratitude for Carlen's journey and skillful retelling of that journey. Gratitude and wisdom are the gifts I predict readers will receive from this book.

Therefore, I urge those of you who are reading this foreword now to move into the maze and the mystery that is Carlen's story, which may also lead you into deeper reflection on the maze and mystery of your own story.

Rev. Dr. Arthur Ross III
Winter 2015

REV. DR. ARTHUR ROSS III is an ordained minister who served churches in New York, Florida, and North Carolina. Dr. Ross is pastor emeritus of White Memorial Presbyterian Church in Raleigh, North Carolina, retiring in 2009 after fifteen years there. He is the former chair of the board of trustees at Union Presbyterian Seminary in Richmond, Virginia, and he continues to be involved in a variety of national and international ministries.

A NIGHTMARE LAID BARE

In a life of wholeness we may face brokenness and
endure woundedness, but our suffering will not be
meaningless. Meaningless suffering is soul-destroying.

—Archbishop Desmond Tutu and Mpho Tutu,
*Made for Goodness: And Why This Makes
All the Difference*

I had a recurring nightmare as a boy. I dreamed I was riding a
bike when I slammed into an invisible wall. I always survived
this crash without injury. But after waking up in a cold sweat,
I was left asking these questions: Why can't I see the wall? Can
someone show me how to avoid that wall? Why am I feeling so
lonely?

These were much the same questions I asked when my wife
Martha ran headlong into an invisible wall called Alzheimer's.
She was diagnosed with this disease in 1997 at age fifty. I didn't

see the wall up ahead. Neither did Martha. We never expected it; we never had a clue. And never had we felt so abandoned and alone. Little did I realize how dramatically our life together was about to change.

The story I'm telling is about a young family's sudden shift from a comfortable, middle-class American life into an alien world shaped and defined by this insidious disease. Though we were forced to face this disease, our story isn't just about Alzheimer's. You or a loved one may be staring at your own crisis—cancer, stroke, job loss, diabetes, heart attack, home foreclosure—you name it. Regardless of the crisis, the potential for emotional and psychological upheaval—alienation, depression, fear, anxiety attacks, a cold numbness—is much the same for victim and family, for care-receiver and caregiver.

But this is not a story about hopelessness. Rather, our story traces a different path that emerged during our family's darkest hours, a path that we did not foresee. Encouraged by a Protestant minister and friend, just after the diagnosis, Martha and I drove from our home in Florida to visit a Catholic nun in Kentucky. This path first appeared among the hills and back roads there.

As we were drawn into this twisting journey, I scrambled for answers. In the months and years that followed, I devoured scores of books, flew halfway around the world to Australia, spent dozens of weekends at a monastery near our home, and found myself all alone one week in Thomas Merton's cabin. In my search I discovered a place far more real than any crisis. I think Martha did too, for this path eventually led us to a ground that transcends any debilitating disease. How it emerged is still a mystery to me.

Perhaps the answer can be found in the statement, "Seek and you will find."

In telling our story, I must speak in Christian terms and images because that's the faith and tradition I grew up with, carried into adulthood, and, after a long drought, embraced. In doing this I'm not denying another's spiritual heritage. Our story is not about scoring theological points. It's about trying to survive, about finding what works and what doesn't as we move through a dark, inscrutable maze. It's about stepping outside our comfort zone to reach anything that holds fast and true. Words do matter. But the truth behind the words matters more.

Some people are just not into spiritual issues. I get that. I've been there too, even though I considered myself Christian. So if you're not, you may want to put this book down now because this is where it's heading—into the spiritual. The names God and Jesus Christ are overused today, and are often abused for manipulative reasons, so any sane person might pause before invoking them out in the public square. Yet here's my dilemma: I can't tell our story without calling on their names, often in the most intimate of ways.

A Search Begins

Before I get too far into our story, I need to share with you who Martha was during the first twenty-five years of our marriage, before she was diagnosed with Alzheimer's. Two traits describe her best: passionate and confident. She loved our three children and her many friends. She loved politics and the numerous civic involvements in which she took a leadership role, especially when she worked with disenfranchised children and families. But Martha was not all work. She loved to dance and play tennis and do almost anything outdoors. And through all these endeavors, she loved her God.

Not long after we moved to St. Petersburg in 1975 and our first child, David, was born, Martha helped manage the local campaign for Jimmy Carter's first presidential run. She soon co-managed a first-time state legislative campaign for a friend who subsequently rose to be Florida's Speaker of the House. She worked with another friend who won a seat on our city council. And Martha worked locally on Lawton Chiles's successful bid for governor of Florida. Martha also was elected to St. Petersburg's city council, serving six years in the 1980s. That council made a number of controversial, big-dollar decisions, the ramifications of which are still felt today—in a significantly good way, I think. Meantime, I was intent on getting into the newspaper business and finally landed a job with the award-winning *St. Petersburg Times* (now *Tampa Bay Times*), where I worked for several years as a journalist before leaving to launch my regional business magazine.

When we got the news that Martha had Alzheimer's, my reporter instincts kicked in. Neither she nor I was used to encountering problems with no solutions. So I ran down a lot of rabbit trails looking for answers to one question: is there any way to get out of this Alzheimer's thing?

Some of these trails proved helpful while others led nowhere. Sometimes I hit a wall and broke through it. Other times I hit a wall and broke my heart. In reporting our story, I describe events that have occurred over seventeen years, from the time of Martha's diagnosis until her death. Yet, unlike a traditional journalist, I also report on events that arose within the subterranean reaches of my heart and mind.

From Journal to Book

This book almost didn't happen. Early on, Rev. Lacy Harwell, a mentor and friend to both Martha and me, wrote on a Christmas card: "Have you considered keeping a journal? It could be of great value to others. As I ponder your notes to me, I feel like a student in a post-grad seminar on love and care. Whatever else you are doing, you are instructing me." I already had begun a journal, but Lacy's urging cemented my commitment, which resulted in fourteen volumes written through the first decade of Martha's illness. This journal gathered dust for five or six years until I decided to crack it open and piece together our story. As I reread it, I thought to myself: *Oh, this is raw*. Old wounds reopened on almost every page as I was reminded of the slow, relentless march of Alzheimer's. *I don't know if I can tell this story*, I thought. I finally started thinking about all we went through and decided our story was worth telling.

If you tease apart the threads, you'll see experiences that brim with bitterness, frustration, rage, guilt, fear, and futility. But you should also see and feel relief, humor, joy, mercy, trust, healing, and gratitude. Our story told here is gleaned from memories, journal entries, epiphanies, poems, prayers, and songs that reveal our family's spirit, splintered and broken— and then recollected and reshaped into a wholeness we could not have imagined.

As I share our story, I must refer to Alzheimer's disease and describe its impact on our family. However, with all due respect to Dr. Alois Alzheimer, who identified this specific dementia a century ago, the name of this disease doesn't deserve the respect conferred by its capitalization. Therefore, from this point forward I will refer to it as . . . *alzheimer's.*

I also need to make one more thing very clear: While we walked along this spiritual path that unfolded before Martha and me, we stayed in close communication with Martha's neurologist. We went to all of Martha's scheduled appointments. Martha took all the medications he prescribed, primarily for the symptoms of alzheimer's and for the seizures that occurred later. We enrolled Martha in an experimental program that he supervised, but which proved unsuccessful. I consider our relationship with Martha's neurologist to have been professional and empathetic, and vital to what we were trying to do.

PART ONE

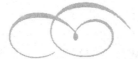

MARTHA, ME, AND THE MONASTICS

ONE

(HEART) BREAKING NEWS

For the thing that I fear comes upon me,
and what I dread befalls me.
—Job 3:25

Our World Is Shaken

September 23, 1997. The date is seared in my mind. That day we were scheduled for a follow-up visit with the doctor who had run some tests on my wife, Martha. Two months earlier, Martha had gone alone for those tests, but she had walked out of the doctor's office before even meeting with him. "I got tired of waiting," she said. That was it, no other explanation—end of subject.

The previous eighteen months had been tough on Martha. She had run for Florida's state legislature as a favored candidate and lost. Then there was the car accident, in which she bumped her head. And other stressful issues related to her health—first a D&C, then two detached retinas. Weird things.

Martha grew lethargic following that political loss, which was so unlike her. Her energy level always was twice mine. Her style had been to bounce back and leap forward. She thought fast, moved fast, laughed loud, and then asked, "What's next?" Rarely was there a dull moment, and if there was, Martha made sure it didn't last long. But now she was checking off fewer items from her long list of things to do. And I heard her laughing less and less on the phone with her buddies.

So in the summer of 1997, nine months after that election loss, the children and I wanted to get to the bottom of her listless attitude. Martha did too. But then, she didn't. I went with her for the rescheduled appointment in early September. The neurologist had set up a series of tests that day—memory, psychological, and neurological, plus blood work.

"Forgetfulness could be due to one of several short-term conditions," the doctor told us. *That sounds encouraging,* I thought.

These tests were designed to screen for various possibilities— amnesia, depression, brain infection, and exhaustion. But I also thought it could be much worse, and I suspected Martha did too.

The next couple of weeks crept at a snail's pace as we awaited the test results. We tried to act busy—I at the magazine and Martha around the house and spending time with her friends. I can't remember looking into Martha's eyes during those two long weeks. I was afraid of what I might find.

Finally, the day for the follow-up appointment arrived. At the medical clinic, Martha and I took the elevator up a couple of floors to the neurologist's office. "Hi, this is Martha Maddux, and I'm her husband," I said to the attendant at the front desk. "We're here for my wife's test results." Martha normally would have been fully capable of speaking for herself, but this long wait had taken its toll.

We sat holding hands and whispering to each other, talking about anything that helped relieve the tension. I gazed around the office, which was little different from any other doctor's office. After several long minutes, the attendant looked our way and said, "Ms. Maddux." We went to the window together, still holding hands. "I'm sorry, but the doctor had an emergency and was called away. One of his associates will be meeting with you, and he's ready to see you."

I paused, disconcerted by this news. Martha and I had warmed to the neurologist at our first appointment, and we expected to see him again. My eyes connected long enough with Martha's to see her concern. But we had little time to react as the attendant directed us straightaway into the associate's office.

This doctor, rather stiff and formal, invited us in and immediately sat behind his big desk while waving us to seats opposite him. I don't remember if we even shook hands or said hello. Social skills apparently weren't a priority for him. He could have been a perfect stand-in for Mr. Spock on *Star Trek*.

Could this be starting off any worse? I wondered.

I found out soon enough. With no introduction, the doctor looked straight at Martha and said, "I'm sorry to tell you this, but it appears likely that you have early onset alzheimer's disease." His voice was calm, ice-cold calm. His words were harsh beyond belief, freezing our hearts and minds.

With this pronouncement, Martha and I looked at each other in pained bewilderment. Her blue eyes instantly dulled as her confident bearing crumbled. She seemed to have retreated into her shadow. Me? Who knows where I went. Maybe into Dante's fifth circle of hell. Our world wasn't turned upside down. It was imploding before our eyes.

"Are you sure—alzheimer's?" I asked, desperate. "Surely there's some mistake."

"No, there's no mistake," said the doctor, who then started to explain the technical processes and probabilities behind the testing procedures.

As though we care, I thought. *Just get us out of here. This can't be happening to Martha. Isn't this disease something you worry about when you get old?* Martha had turned fifty only twenty days earlier, the same day that I had turned fifty-two.

We slipped out of the doctor's office confused and dazed, hand clutching hand, two shadows fleeing. Making our way home, a silent fury of questions was unleashed within me, one piled up on the other: *Why was Martha hit with this? She's bright, she's engaging, and she's a go-getter. How do we tell our children? How will they handle this? What will Martha's family think? Her friends? Who can we turn to for answers? Are there any answers? Oh God—help!*

Martha and I felt trapped in a dark place with no way out. The medical community says alzheimer's is a degenerative disease of the brain that has no known cause or cure. Yet after recovering from the initial shock, my first instinct was to prove the doctors wrong.

I must have read a hundred books, pamphlets, or articles in short order. And anything I felt Martha could learn from, I shared with her. Probably the best book we read together was *Alzheimer's Disease: Frequently Asked Questions* by Frena Gray-Davidson, a professional caregiver. I quickly learned from her that my number-one priority as Martha's caregiver, if I wanted to be useful for the long haul, was to take care of myself. Easier said than done, I discovered, for the verdict we'd been handed was ugly and fatalistic, consuming all my energy and attention. We were two flies caught in a spider's web, ready to be picked apart piece by piece.

Shocks, Aftershocks, and More Shocks

Prior to this, our lives had begun orbiting into something of a sweet spot. Martha and I had been married twenty-five years. Our three kids were approaching young adulthood without any of us showing too many scars. So we had more time for pursuits other than parenting. Martha had always enjoyed her civic activities, including her time on our city council. She was known for her direct questions and comments; in fact, she was too pointed at times, critics said. Martha turned out to be the swing vote on one of the city's most controversial issues ever—whether to build a $100 million baseball stadium when they had no major league team to fill it. It's now home to the Tampa Bay Rays.

Martha and I had run into plenty of roadblocks in our endeavors, and we stumbled through our share of mistakes. Through them all, though, we were able to recover. But this diagnosis overwhelmed me. I could see no way around it, over it, or through it. I wanted to ignore this crisis but couldn't. Everywhere we turned this thing called alzheimer's shadowed us.

It even followed us onto the tennis courts, where we had always enjoyed playing together. As she had been in most things, Martha was competitive in tennis. But now her smart forehand shots had lost their zing. Her hustle in covering the court was turning into a shuffle. No longer did she want to keep score and win. "Let's just hit," she said.

At my work, our regional business magazine was enjoying a measure of success as it expanded in a competitive media market. But I couldn't focus on the business at hand. I sifted through my in-basket, glanced at the day's deposit, signed checks, made a few calls, and scanned my ten-page to-do list before setting it aside. *Time to go home,* I said, walking away from my desk. As for trying to manage and grow the magazine that I'd started thirteen years earlier, I now let our publisher worry about that.

We began to review our commitments. "Carlen," Martha said and hesitated. "Carlen . . . do you think I should resign?" She was chair of the Juvenile Welfare Board, a county agency that worked with a large number of service organizations for children and families. I didn't know how to respond. I didn't want to pull the rug out from under her. We laid out the pros and cons and any encroaching limitations for handling that job.

"I guess I'd better tell Jim and see what he thinks," Martha whispered. A tear wet her cheek. Jim Mills was the board's executive director. When they talked, the two decided it was best for her to step down as chair while remaining on the board. That decision, though thoughtfully made, still hurt Martha deeply.

This and many other incidences made me realize that the initial shock from the diagnosis was only the first of many. A disease like alzheimer's—or any other devastating crisis—precipitates a whole series of aftershocks, both immediate and long-term. Some people may describe such shocks as emotional and psychological. But that's only partly true. These shocks affected us at a much deeper level, down in a murky realm we call spiritual—threatening to destroy the very core of our existence.

I tried my best to be Martha's anchor. This crisis forced both of us to slow down. It also forced me to be attentive. Before we married, I remember well the time Martha asked me the color of her eyes, and I didn't know. *Oops.* That forced me to be more attentive, but nothing like this crisis did. We started doing more activities together and talking more with each other. And we began to appreciate each other in ways that we'd never realized before.

It's better to be lost together than alone, I decided.

Both Martha and I grew up in Protestant Christian families. We invited Jesus into our lives as our personal Lord and Savior. We were baptized, we took Communion, and we went to church regularly. Yet church was one activity among many in our busy lives. In the days following the diagnosis, Martha and I doubled down on our faith. We prayed and read the Bible together in a way that we'd rarely done. But as we did, I found the words of Scripture to be drier than the paper they were written on. Prayers froze on my lips. And Sunday worship was a mere rind of itself, any juice long squeezed out. All I could do was cry or stare into space. Martha too.

An anxious stream of chatter arose within me: *Where's God in all this? Where's the love? Where's the help? Where's the protection?* In some deep, inarticulate place I began to feel that Martha and I were not loved by God; that he didn't care about our devastating dilemma. And I was too afraid of God to voice that out loud, or to call him out on it. I began to wonder, *If my faith is no good in a crisis like this, then what good is my faith?* I soon discovered that the faith I had built over a lifetime was pretty thin gruel.

A JOURNAL BEGINS

The journal I started shortly after Martha's diagnosis became a gathering place for the information, thoughts, feelings, questions, and observations that were hurtling at me from all angles. I soon realized it also could help me keep our children informed about what was going on and what I was thinking. They needed to know that I was, like them, hurt and confused with few if any answers, but still searching. These are excerpts from my first frantic entries in September 1997.

Our world is turned upside down. On October 7 we'll become part of an experimental study our doctor is participating in. Drug "L" is thought to retard, if not stop, a.d.'s progress.

Martha and I are sharing prayers, crying more than praying.

Martha does NOT want to tell the family yet. I agree. Not until we've absorbed the shock and begun to move in a more positive direction.

I'm seeing a distancing by Kathryn. She doesn't know why her mommie can't think straight or remember. As a result, she writes off Martha's opinions, orders, etc. She needs to know about the diagnosis sooner than either David or Rachel since she's here day-in, day-out.

Martha needs comfort; support; leadership and direction; stress relief; a better understanding of alzheimer's; a strong, trusting relationship with our doctor; spiritual counseling; love, hope, and more of God in her life.

I need time, a focus, support, a better understanding of a.d., a stronger relationship with Jesus. De-stress, de-compress.

TWO PROTESTANTS IN A CATHOLIC MOTHERHOUSE

You must stop examining spiritual truths like dry bones!
You must break open the bones and take in the
life-giving marrow.

—Sadhu Sundar Singh,
Essential Writings

A Question of Willingness

Early in our marriage, before children and between jobs, Martha and I flipped our car on the Alaska Highway. Driving on what must have been the longest gravel road in the world, Martha lost control on a curve with an oil tanker fast approaching. The truck passed, our left tires dropped off the edge of the gravel embankment, and our car performed a perfect midair flip before landing on its roof. *Smack!* Neither of us was injured, suffering not even a scratch as we hung upside down suspended by our seat belts. Her shoulder-length brown hair was dangling straight down, blond highlights and all. We looked at each other wide-eyed, then released our seat belts and slipped out the windows.

Martha's diagnosis felt much the same. Our lives were suspended upside down and shaken. However, we could see no window to slip out to safety. That's why, three weeks after the diagnosis, we found ourselves driving up to Kentucky to visit a Catholic nun we'd never heard of before.

We decided to go at the urging of Rev. Lacy Harwell, our mentor. We had called him soon after the news. He was the Presbyterian minister in St. Petersburg who married us, baptized two of our children, and was Martha's longtime friend. He listened to our story with a focus I'd seen in only a handful of other people. Lacy's whole body was zeroed in on everything we said and felt. The three of us sat downstairs in our living room, Martha and I on a couch and Lacy on a chair opposite. At Martha's request, I described to Lacy what we knew, and she filled in the details that she felt like sharing. A calm soon descended on us all. Lacy's shoulders sagged, and tears crept down the face of this big bear of a man whom I'd never seen cry. I swapped seats with Lacy and let these two friends hug.

Then he told us about his friend and confidant Sr. Elaine Prevallet. "A number of my friends faced with a serious crisis have gone to visit Elaine," Lacy said in a tone so hushed that I could hardly hear him. His voice usually boomed with a rich South Carolina drawl. "I've never met another person with Elaine's gift of discernment. I don't know where your visit might lead, but it would be worth your time and effort."

A couple of weeks and eight hundred miles later, Martha and I showed up at Sr. Elaine's doorstep, not knowing what to expect but hoping desperately to find help. Sr. Elaine was the spiritual director for the retreat center of the Sisters of Loretto, an hour or so south of Louisville. As we approached the entrance to the motherhouse, we passed the half a dozen storefronts that make up the village of Nerinx. Down the road from the Sisters of Loretto is a provider of a different sort of spirit, the Maker's Mark bourbon distillery.

We arrived late in the afternoon, and Sr. Elaine showed us our room and where we would eat. Neither she nor her sisters wore the traditional habit of my stereotyped nun, but just regular street clothes and work clothes. Founded a couple of hundred years ago, Loretto is a community of nuns devoted to education, social justice, and women's issues. The sisters take their religious vows seriously, but unquestioned submission is not numbered among those commitments. These women were vital, independent thinkers.

My first, and lasting, impression of Sr. Elaine was of her eyes. I can't tell you their color, but I do know they are dark and penetrating. Penetrating not in a "Let me find out all your secrets" sort of way, but in a kind, deeply comforting sense. The peace and trust Sr. Elaine conveyed was clear from the start. Her eyes danced with humor and compassion. Her presence in our lives offered a welcome refuge from the worry and uncertainty churning within Martha and me.

We quickly fell into a routine. In the mornings, we spent an hour talking with Sr. Elaine. The rest of the day we either walked or stayed in our room. The Loretto motherhouse is set on an eight-hundred-acre farm, with plenty of room for Martha and me to wander and talk. The trees were ablaze with their October colors. For hours on end, we sat on a bench by a pond, holding hands, discussing our conversations with Sr. Elaine, fighting back tears, wondering how best to tell our children. Although we'd shared the news with Kathryn, our teenager at home, we had yet to tell David or Rachel, who were away at college.

During our week's visit, Martha and I had conversations along two tracks. One was sorting through information from the give-and-take with Sr. Elaine. The other arose out of Martha's desperate desire to answer correctly the questions given to her when she was tested for alzheimer's. We had an upcoming appointment with a second neurologist, and Martha wanted to be ready. She was intent on proving the doctor's diagnosis wrong. And so was I. Such questions were based less on prep work and more on general awareness, yet if Martha wanted to study for these questions, I didn't want to discourage her. Her confidence had suffered enough. So in the privacy of our room, Martha had me quiz her: Who's the President of the United States? When's your birthday? What's today's date? And then there was that arithmetic question that had stumped Martha: start at 100 and subtract by seven, giving the numbers in descending order. Martha had reached ninety-three and could go no further. Because she seemed unable to work out the formula in her mind, Martha wanted to memorize the answer: *100, 93, 86, 79, 72,* and so on.

All this memory work went slowly. Three steps forward, two back; two steps forward, one back. Nonetheless, Martha progressed. She began to get more questions right than wrong. I don't remember how far down the arithmetic scale she got, but she went well beyond ninety-three. However, if we took a break for more than two days, the results of the memory work evaporated. Martha insisted on starting over. And so we did. But it felt like trying to plow through a parched, sunbaked field.

During our early conversations with Sr. Elaine, she listened to our fears and grief, asking a question here and there. She projected a confident humility, like a practical and perceptive mother. Her graying hair was pulled back, framing a face that easily shifted from an expression of compassion to one full of wit and laughter. Her voice had a quiet, gracious authority that could call out your bluff.

Sr. Elaine gently yet firmly began to point out a trait she saw in both Martha and me, of which neither of us had been aware. "You might want to explore the difference between *willfulness* and *willingness*," she said. Sr. Elaine only hinted at what she was thinking and then referred us to a book in their small library called *Will and Spirit* by Gerald G. May, MD. The book was no help; apparently my entrenched mind-set kept me from understanding the author's message.

Our comfortable, middle-class background didn't seem much different from those of our friends and peers. We were busy raising a young family while working hard to succeed in our chosen fields. Politics and running a small, growing business are by definition willful enterprises. *So what's wrong with that?* I wondered. I tried to understand this distinction drawn by Sr. Elaine, but to no avail. My questioning did little but churn up waves of anxiety.

Martha and the Monk

Halfway through our visit, I mentioned to Sr. Elaine my budding interest in Thomas Merton and his insights into meditation. A social activist and prolific writer, Merton had lived at the nearby Abbey of Gethsemani for three decades until his untimely death in 1968.

Sr. Elaine suggested we attend Gethsemani's evening Compline service. It's the last of several daily prayer services. She also said we might want to stay afterward for the short talk usually given by Fr. Matthew Kelty. He had been a close friend of Merton's, Sr. Elaine said. That raised the level of my curiosity several more notches. Martha said she was willing to go, but I could tell she was reluctant as the slightest change in place and people was becoming an issue.

On a late Tuesday afternoon, we drove the dozen or so miles to Gethsemani, winding through the rolling countryside marked by its bright, wooded hills, or *knobs,* as they're called there. From afar, the monastery's tiled roofs, white walls, and fortresslike compound reminded me of a medieval castle or cathedral. Several buildings outlined the horizon, but one in the middle towered above the others. *That must be the sanctuary*, I thought when seeing it.

Inside the church, the ceiling towered three stories above. Guests sat toward the front entrance while the monks, in their black-and-white robes, slipped silently into the center of the narrow nave and took their designated seats—half on one side and half on the other, facing each other. I found the newness of it all intriguing—new to me, that is.

When the brothers bowed in prayer, we bowed. When Scriptures were read, we listened. When the monks chanted the Psalms back and forth from one side to the other, we tried to sing. But the trappings of the place attracted me more than the service. *So this is where Thomas Merton worshiped,* I thought, with a trace of childish awe. *I wonder where he sat.* I then remembered a story Merton told regarding their rule of silence. Trappist practices and vows are among the strictest of Catholic monastic orders. To communicate without breaking their silence, Merton and a handful of comrades had developed something akin to a Morse code—a *tap-tap-tap* here and a quick *tap-tap* there. As I sat in the pew, I had to catch myself from laughing out loud at the whimsical scene playing out in my mind.

After the service, Martha and I walked out the front entrance, immediately turning left into a smaller room along with a couple dozen other folks this night. Fr. Matthew Kelty shuffled in and began to talk. I was instantly drawn to him and his message while wondering about Martha's reaction. I never knew with whom she would feel comfortable, given her current state of mind. After his homily, Martha and I and the other guests remained seated while Fr. Matthew slipped out.

On our drive along the dark country road back to Loretto, Martha surprised me when I asked her how she liked the service. "I want to go back," she said without hesitation. Thus we did the next evening. The following excerpt from my journal gives an added sense of why Martha and I were drawn to Fr. Matthew.

OCTOBER 22, 1997

He's one of the most incisive Christian pundits I've heard. He riveted his audience with a swift opening round of poetry and Scripture, followed by off-the-cuff comments and a side dish of wisecracks. His spontaneous delivery, frumpish appearance, and crusty confidence announced we were in the presence of a curmudgeon, a South Boston Irish one at that. Fr. Matthew, who's in his early eighties, is grounded in a robust faith and a passion for poetry. I've encountered few others who have his way with words. His humor strikes dead center—not to destroy, only to provoke. At the end of his homily, I didn't know whether to laugh or cry.

After his homily the second night, Fr. Matthew again exited behind us, but he didn't get five steps before Martha bolted from her seat and walked straight up to him. The two spoke briefly, and then as Fr. Matthew continued to make his way to the door, Martha turned back to join me. A smile played across her lips; her eyes were bright with excitement.

"What was that about?" I asked.

"I told him about my alzheimer's," she said.

"And . . . ?"

"And he said, 'Come and see me tomorrow at two-thirty.'"

On Thursday, then, we drove for the third consecutive day along the now-familiar road to Gethsemani. We went to the library, where Fr. Matthew was waiting. His stooped shoulders and lined face gave him an air of worldly weariness, yet his faint smile and red cheeks, almost elfin-like, showed no sense of despair.

His dark eyes greeted us kindly. "Hello, Martha. This must be your husband."

Martha smiled shyly and looked my way.

"Hello, Fr. Matthew. I'm Carlen," I said as we shook hands.

"I'm pleased to meet you," he said. "Perhaps it would be all right, Carlen, if Martha and I spoke alone? Would you be willing to leave us for an hour?"

His request caught me off guard, for I'd expected the three of us to talk together. I quickly looked at Martha, and she easily nodded *yes*. I was okay with that as long as she was. They walked into his office, and I wondered, *What am I going to do now?*

Gethsemani conveys a sense of mystery. It's one of the oldest monasteries in the United States, and the first one I'd visited. As I explored the grounds, a delicious irony occurred to this kid from a family of religious teetotalers: while the monastery is grounded in disciplines of silence, work, and prayer, it is much better known for its bourbon-soaked fudges and fruitcakes.

After an hour of poking my head in and out of buildings, gazing at a cemetery in search of Merton's gravesite, and just sitting quietly, I returned to the library where Martha and Fr. Matthew were waiting. The following journal entry recounts the visit.

OCTOBER 23, 1997

There in the library, Fr. Matthew told Martha and me that suffering and illness offer no easy answer for why they occur. "This is now a spiritual journey," he said.

"Don't go bitter; draw on faith's deepest strength. Drink deep from God's well; it's his gift."

He looked straight into Martha's eyes. "You came calling on me," he said. "You are now one of us. So from now on, you are in my prayer."

He suggested that when Martha returned home she set aside a time for silence away from the house, in a favorite church or solitary spot. He also told Martha to take one of the abbey's Psalters and use it as a devotional. The Psalter is the book of Psalms set to music akin to a Gregorian chant.

After Fr. Matthew left, Martha had difficulty explaining to me all that was said during their private conversation. But I could tell that whatever it was, it was meaningful. For the first time in weeks, Martha's face appeared relaxed. She carried herself with an air of confidence, as though she were saying, "I know something that you don't." Her eyes were as clear and blue as I've ever seen. Martha called Fr. Matthew "my new friend."

Martha and I had only seen Gethsemani at night before that day, and it was a pretty, fall afternoon, so we decided to walk. Across the road were woods, part of the monastery's two thousand acres. High on a knob to the left stood a large white cross, its massive arms open wide. *A welcome sign maybe, inviting us or anyone else who feels abandoned?*

On reaching the woods' edge, we saw a path and took it. There was nothing unique about this path; what was different was Martha—she was bouncing along the path with a confidence I thought I would never see again. At times she led; other times she stopped to inspect a rock or a wildflower. And with every sun-speckled step, the autumn leaves seemed brighter than usual, while the rocks and roots and wood ferns expressed a quiet joy that I'd not experienced on a walk before or since.

The woods were thick enough that, despite the bright afternoon sun, the trail was dark as we walked it. At the top of the knob, the woods opened onto a sunlit cow pasture, rich and green. There were no cows this day, only three or four deer gathered in the distance. We looked at them, and the deer looked at us. Then they turned back to face each other as though they were holding some council meeting. We turned back down the path. When we reached bottom, Martha stepped down to a dry creek bed. She picked up three small stones that fit into her palm. "In the name of the Father, the Son, and the Spirit," we said as Martha folded her fingers over the stones. We walked back to our car and drove to Loretto.

Two days after that walk in Gethsemani, and after Martha's visit with Fr. Matthew, we left Sr. Elaine and the Loretto community for home. During one of our last conversations, Sr. Elaine suggested that we check out alternative forms of medicine and that we look further into the practice of meditation. We had come to Loretto frightened and disheartened; we left feeling more secure. We had come confused; we left more focused. We had come unsure what to do or where to go; we left sensing a path opening before us. The chaos within us was subsiding. I was still anxious about Martha's condition, but my anxiety was greatly reduced, as Martha's also appeared to be.

We both felt we had guides we could call on in Fr. Matthew and Sr. Elaine. As we parted, Sr. Elaine spoke these last words to us: "Your main calling at this time is to trust that you belong to God and not to yourselves. And to deepen your love for God and between yourselves."

We should be able to do that, I remember thinking.

THREE

SMOKE SIGNALS FROM A MONASTERY

Fold the wings of your mind. Place your mind in your
heart. Come into the presence of God.

—Ancient Eastern Orthodox verse,
shared by Sr. Elaine Prevallet

"Martha, we need to talk," I said after we had run some
errands together.

"Talk about what?" She turned to look at me as she set a
couple of bags down on the kitchen table.

I hesitated. I wrapped both my hands around Martha's,
saying, "I'm afraid you've got to stop driving."

The pressure to stop driving had been building since her
diagnosis three years earlier. I'd let Martha drive the car despite

the doctor's strong warning. I didn't have the nerve then to make her stop.

Martha's blue eyes froze. She pulled her hands away. "Why?" she spat back.

"Don't you realize you ran a red light fifteen minutes ago?"

"What red light?"

"That's my point, Martha. You're missing things when you drive. You could have a bad wreck and hurt yourself or someone else."

Martha's face flushed. She tried to state her position, but her words were scrambled. We gazed at each other. I was dumbstruck. I didn't know what else to say to help her see the potential danger of her driving. Her glazed, sad eyes told me she felt I'd betrayed her. Martha turned her back, paused, and then ran upstairs to our bedroom without saying another word.

I pulled the keys from her purse, grabbed the extra ones from the key rack, and hid them in a desk drawer. Then I walked straight into the bathroom downstairs, slammed the door shut, and sat on the floor, numb. I was unsure what hurt most—having to take the keys away or being forced to hear my usually articulate wife argue her case in a fumbling, halting manner.

I didn't just take her keys away, I cried. *I cut out Martha's heart.*

Not since the news of Martha's diagnosis had I felt this devastated. An old demon called despair was rearing its ugly head, and this puzzled me. *Haven't I made any progress at all? It never stops, does it? This alzheimer's disease keeps coming at us. Just when it feels as if we've reached solid ground, it turns to quicksand.*

A Funny Thing Happened on My Way to Peace, Tranquility, and Enlightenment

Until this car-key incident, a measure of peace had settled over Martha and me. The uncertainty of our uneven life had seemed a bit steadier the past three years as we practiced meditation at Sr. Elaine's encouragement.

After we returned from her retreat center, I asked Rev. Lacy Harwell what he knew about meditation. I said I had read Merton's book on contemplative prayer, but found it to be complicated. Lacy said Sr. Elaine introduced him to meditation as a possible help for his high blood pressure. "I practiced a few days with her and actually saw my pressure drop," he boasted. "Then Elaine told me, 'That's good. Now let's see if you're disciplined enough to meditate the rest of your life.'" Lacy burst out with that full-throated laugh of his. I hadn't met a Protestant Christian, let alone a minister, who practiced a contemplative form of prayer. "Catholics have a rich heritage of this," Lacy said. "Protestants don't."

My earlier readings of meditation had left me feeling furtive, almost heretical. Although Transcendental Meditation had arrived on the scene in the 1960s, many middle-of-the-road Christians in 1997 still considered meditation in any form to be a Far Eastern mystery. Even so, I rather enjoyed being out on the edge of this "heresy." Talking with Lacy gave me permission to explore further.

Little was conventional about Lacy. After four decades of active ministry, he retired in 1995, whereupon he learned to drive big rig trucks. He shed his coat and tie and minister's frock from his six-foot-four, 265-pound frame and stepped into a pair of overalls, a work shirt, and size-thirteen farm boots. Lacy went to work hauling seed and fertilizer for his family's farm outside Florence, South Carolina. This truck hauler is the same man who years earlier earned advanced degrees from Princeton Theological Seminary, the University of Edinburgh, and Union Theological Seminary in New York, where he studied under the likes of Reinhold Niebuhr.

As we discussed meditation, Lacy told us to check out a Benedictine monk named John Main, the developer of a contemplative practice called Christian Meditation. "He's the best I've found. He's really good at making meditation understandable to the average person." With Main's method, you silently repeat a prescribed word for twenty to thirty minutes in the morning and evening. "There are a few other guidelines," Lacy said, "but that's basically it."

That's simple enough, I thought. I went online in search of Fr. John Main and ordered his book *Word into Silence* and a set of tapes called *In the Beginning*. When the package arrived, Martha and I read the book together and listened to the tapes. I became more comfortable when I learned that John Main had traced this form of prayer back to the early years of Christianity, to the Desert Fathers of the fourth century.

As Martha and I meditated, we sat side by side on the living-room couch, holding hands. I whispered the word that we'd selected, because I was unsure whether Martha was able to repeat it to herself. After several weeks I asked her, "Is this helping?"

"I think so," she said, unable to explain further. Martha did appear more relaxed and less confused. And that made me less desperate. We had learned to expect no clear answers in this twilight zone called alzheimer's. Yet out of these shared moments a bond of silence arose between us. *This is different,* I thought. We had done a lot of things together—walking, talking, watching TV, reading the paper and the Bible, screaming at each other, playing tennis—but in our twenty-five years of marriage we had not sat together for any period of meaningful silence. *This is really good.* We hadn't known this depth of intimacy in any other setting, even in bed.

For most of our marriage, Martha had been the one more spiritually committed. And her conviction carried forward into this crisis. After returning from Kentucky, Martha drove each day to a chapel downtown to sit quietly in the sanctuary. She took a well-worn Bible and the Psalter given her by Fr. Matthew. Martha had difficulty sharing what occurred during these moments, but I could sense the calm gathering within her.

Meanwhile, I also felt a need to meditate by myself, which I did in the early morning and evening. When I started, I thought that once I was into the swing of meditation, an unceasing peace would bubble up from some deep well. I did sense a quantum of silence and rest. But after several months, the more I practiced this contemplative form of prayer, the more an overwhelming sense of discouragement stirred within me.

I'm making no progress whatsoever, I thought. *This is one step forward and ten back. Why bother?*

Yet John Main encouraged us through his book and audiotapes to keep going. He emphasizes three points throughout—perseverance, patience, and being attentive. These are vital for meditation to yield lasting results. In meditation, Main says in *Word into Silence,* "we seek not to think about God, but to be with God, to experience Him as the ground of our being."

I decided to soldier on, at least for a while. As I did, meditation helped me peer into my heart and mind, and when I saw more clearly what was there, all hell broke loose.

The memory is still vivid. Images of bird wings by the score flapping against the panes of my mind. *Breathe in*—wings of fear flapping; *breathe out*—wings of anxiety. Anxiety upon fear, circling from above and below, diving at me, and attacking me: *flap-flap-flap-flap-flap-flap-flap-flap-flap-flap!*

God! What is going on?

These dark wings are trying to destroy me.

Breathe in, slowly. Breathe out, slowly. Keep saying your word, Carlen. Breathe in; breathe out. At all costs, hold on to your word.

Is this what they felt like in the Hitchcock film, The Birds? *Have I repressed my feelings that much? Jesus!* I called out, cursing and crying for help in the same breath. *Am I losing my mind? Is this an anxiety attack?*

But this was no anxiety attack, which I know from experience can leave you cowering in a corner. Instead, I felt deeply entrenched anxieties loosening from their moorings. My heart was opening up. I began to worry less. The rising tension I felt from worrying about Martha's symptoms was easing. I was better able to focus on her needs. My focus at work improved. Since that experience, those wings of darkness haven't returned.

Is this what you mean, Sr. Elaine? Is my hard-headed willfulness starting to break up?

The practice of meditative prayer, while simple in form, requires more discipline than I'd imagined. It is so counterintuitive for a guy like me who wants to control his emotions, his environment, and his relationships. *Be still so you can do more.*

Suspend your thinking, Carlen, so your thoughts can come clear. Stop stressing so you can enjoy God enjoying you. Such contrarian ideas had never dawned on me before I started to meditate.

The process of learning to meditate reminds me of when I learned to snow ski. After a thousand spills, I finally realized that skiing works better and is much more fun when I stop trying to control the skis and relax, letting them do the work. Like any new skier, when I started to fall I leaned back into the slope to try to regain my balance. And I always fell. But I finally figured out what the instructor was saying: lean out away from the slope; let your upper body hang out over the slope, and relax. When I leaned out, the edges of my skis were able to cut into the snow and keep me from falling.

New to meditation, I soon realized how easily distracted I am. I tried to control the distractions by shooing them away— or worse, by trying to grip them through the sheer force of my will. Such attempts are futile. And the more I meditated, the more I became aware of the mental and emotional baggage that I'd packed away. Painfully aware. Hiding this baggage was such a natural response, just like leaning back into the ski slope when I started to fall.

But after more than enough pain, I began to realize that I must step aside and let Christ do the work. Let him upend my anxieties; let him cut loose my obsessive, wrongheaded beliefs. With Martha's declining abilities and my magazine's financial pressures, I often felt overwhelmed—a wedge of tension was forming in my head. I was most aware of it during my periods of silence. One day it was intense; the next day it subsided. The pain was acute, and no amount of aspirin made it disappear.

I worried: *Did Mom and Dad have a similar feeling?* Both died from brain cancer. Now that scared me. *God, do I have to worry about this too? On top of Martha's care and my business?*

I kept at the meditation—twenty minutes in the morning and twenty in the evening. *Breathe in; breathe out. Breathe in; breathe out. Let the tension go, Carlen. Be attentive to your word.* In a few weeks, a comforting warmth began to form around this wedge of tension. *This is strange,* I thought. *This feels like the palm of a hand.* In my mind's eye, I could see this hand move the wedge from side to side, loosening bands of worry and fear. Then one day this hand gently lifted the wedge from my head, slowly and surely, as though it were pulling a root from the ground. Any remnant of a headache was gone.

Who Let the Dogs Out?

As I progressed in the practice of meditation, and not long after I took Martha's car keys away, our children gave me a priceless gift. They gave me a weekend a month off for nearly a decade. This was not an easy gift on their part. From late Friday afternoon through Sunday afternoon, they stayed with their mother. As months progressed into years, those weekends included making meals or taking her out to eat, helping her change clothes, and figuring out activities to do together such as taking a walk, playing tennis, going to a movie, visiting a friend, or watching TV. The physical aspects were hard, but the emotional were harder. The reversal of the parent-child role unleashed in our children an emotional undertow that they learned to navigate with a grace far beyond their twenty-something years.

Most of those weekends off I spent at a small Benedictine monastery an hour north of St. Petersburg. I decided to try St. Leo Abbey because of our visits with Sr. Elaine and Fr. Matthew. St. Leo turned out to be a godsend. I found no better place to rant and pour out my anguish and fears. I could have rented a motel room on the beach, but it wouldn't have offered the undistracted silence I needed.

St. Leo gave me the mental and emotional space to digest what I'd been reading and doing and thinking. My mind became more open and relaxed as I meditated and prayed. Much of what I learned about dealing with Martha's symptoms was either initiated or struggled with during these weekends. I learned surprising truths about God and even more surprising truths about myself and my relation to God. This kind of learning is not heady or academic. This is experiential learning at its most basic. I realized that what I think should work often does not.

I recognized that a willing mind can see options to which a fearful, willful mind is blind. A good example: I'm on an afternoon walk near St. Leo, with no cars and only a few houses lining the country road. The only sounds are my shoes crunching on the loose gravel and dogs barking in the distance. I am lost in my thoughts when I realize the barking is getting louder and closer. Out of nowhere two large dogs—a hunting hound and a German shepherd—are charging me. *This is no welcome to the neighborhood.* I run, but they're gaining on me. I pick up some rocks and start throwing. They dodge everything, but do back off. But I run out of rocks and sticks and they start charging back mad, growling and baring their ugly yellow teeth. *This is getting real nasty.*

My heart is racing. *What can I do?* A friend's offbeat idea flashes into my mind. *What have I got to lose?* I take several deep breaths and bow my head, watching the dogs from the corner of my eye, careful not to make eye contact. As they circle, I circle. As they reverse, I reverse. Shaking, I silently affirm: *I'm a creation of God, as you are. You dogs have nothing to fear, just as I have nothing to fear. We are God's creatures, loved and adored by him. He fills you with peace, as he fills me with peace. We cannot harm each other; we care for each other.*

As I repeat this, my heart returns to a more regular beat and my fear subsides. I feel warmth from within, which I've since come to know as God's healing light. As best I can, I let it flow through me. *Please stream through these dogs too.* The dogs back away. *Maybe I can start walking.* I start moving and they charge, snapping at my legs. I stop. *Okay, Carlen, once more: I'm loved as you are loved; I have nothing to fear just as you have nothing to fear.* The dogs back away again. After a long, silent standoff, I hear a whimper and open my eyes. The dogs have turned tail, trotting back to their house. I walk back to St. Leo with one eye over my shoulder, repeating all the way there, *Thank you, Father, thank you.*

For all I know, the dogs grew bored. There's no question, though, that a restful yet alert energy developed within me, and these dogs somehow picked up on it. I don't want to make too much of the incident, but I can say this: repeatedly since then, I have felt a clenched fist of fear in my mind open into a receptive palm of trust.

Is this what you mean by being willing, Sr. Elaine?

What's Love Got to Do with It?

Such moments of willingness were rare in the early days of our journey. Yet they've long remained in my memory. On another weekend at St. Leo, I was praying that alzheimer's be lifted from Martha and our family. As I did, I heard a whisper within me, and I asked, *What are you saying?* I couldn't understand the words, yet their meaning was clear: *Carlen, you don't have to settle for this fractured existence being dished out by alzheimer's.*

That whispered impression startled me. And I exclaimed, *Exactly how in this tragedy do you find anything but a fractured existence?* I complained silently: *I need a consistent, clear direction. Yet everything comes in impressions and whispers and glimpses and winks and fleeting thoughts—everything but the pain.* The pain of seeing Martha slip away was unmistakable and relentless.

Out of this cloud of confusion a faint question emerged. This question had a certain familiarity, as though it had been shadowing me for a lifetime. It often arose in the early morning when Martha was asleep by my side, during that dark stillness when the bats of our minds begin to stir.

Do I believe? No, do I know? Do I know deep within, down where the rawest of memories and fears hide out? Do I know that the Lord my God loves me with all his heart? Do I know that my God loves me with all his soul? With all his strength? And with all his mind?

Answering, "Yes, God loves me," might have been easy when life was good. But it was quite another matter to know and feel that love when much of my world had turned sour and cold, and the only certainty I felt was a numb nothingness.

This question weighed on my heart and mind for weeks

until I felt a vast chasm within me—a hole dug deep by the pain of isolation. God stood on one side; I on the other, engulfed in fear. Most of my life I thought all that was required of me was to believe in God and do what he said to do. But now I faced a hard truth: my faith was a dry, secondhand belief with little depth and less passion. It had been built largely upon what authorities said I should believe and do—authorities such as Moses and Paul from the Bible, my parents and grandparents, preachers, peers, teachers, and writers. I had to admit that I was a practicing Christian largely because of the authority I'd lent to these voices outside me, not because of the authority of a voice and presence within.

As I stood peering into the depths of this chasm, I glimpsed what I'd never seen—the vast difference between *believing in* God and *believing* God. Then *poof!*—the image of this chasm dissolved. My mind went quiet. A drop of something fresh overcame me. *It's the sweetest thing I've ever tasted,* I thought, as peace flooded my mind and body. I'd read enough of the more sublime writings from the Bible and from some saints and mystics to recognize in this their depictions of divine love. *That's what this tastes like; it's the love described in those accounts.*

Then it disappeared.

I want more! I cried out. *How do I taste more of whatever this is—this love? What do I need to do? How can I get across this chasm?*

I wanted to be whole. Not whole *again*, but whole for the first time in my life. I realized that I hadn't felt whole as an adult, as a parent, as a college student, or as a kid. I'd felt confident at school and sports and work, yet as I reflect back, such confidence is better characterized as self-absorption. And that, I've learned, is far from being whole.

Months after feeling this vast chasm in my heart, I met with an older friend who impressed me as being experienced in the ways of things spiritual. "How can I get across this chasm?" I asked him. "How can I find this love that I tasted, this wholeness?"

He told me, "This kind of search can be frustrating and challenging. Even overwhelming." Yet he quickly added, "It also could result in the richest reward you ever receive."

He cautioned me, though, should I continue in this direction: "If you remember nothing else from our conversation, Carlen, remember this: *Be gentle on yourself.*"

I didn't know what he meant at first. *It's pretty easy to take care of myself,* I thought. Reflecting on his admonition now reminds me of something my father taught me when I was a kid. Dad, who owned a hardware store, was showing me how to open a lock with a key. "If it doesn't turn easy, Carlen, don't force it."

Today, as I think back on Dad's advice, I'm reminded of the occasions I've willfully tried to force outcomes I wanted and come too close to destroying things far more valuable than a lock and key—occasions like taking Martha's car keys away. The silent beating I gave myself still hurts, and my friend's forewarning echoes in my mind: *Be gentle on yourself, Carlen; be gentle.*

MY WEEKENDS AT ST. LEO ABBEY

Tampa Bay is a sprawling region with three million people. You wouldn't know St. Leo Abbey lies alongside the region's growth path except for the traffic that blows by on the two-lane highway that cuts St. Leo's property in half. Otherwise, the monastery is as one might expect: quiet, and moving with the rhythm established sixteen centuries ago by St. Benedict. To the left of the abbey church is a small guesthouse where I stay. It nestles up against an orange grove that spills down into a good-sized body of water called Lake Jovita. The canopies of large live oaks offer ample shade throughout the grounds.

Rooms in the guesthouse are spare yet comfortable, each with one or two twin beds, a small desk, a reading chair and lamp, a bath and shower, and an AC window unit. Communal areas include a kitchen, a study room with a small case of books, a sitting area with a TV, and a back porch looking out over the lake.

Typically, I would leave for St. Leo straight from work, usually midafternoon Friday. Martha would remain with her daytime caregiver until one of the children arrived for the evening. My weekend retreats were self-directed, but in a loose way because I would usually arrive with no agenda in mind other than to be still and quiet. They were make-it-up-as-you-go retreats, but I like to think Christ's Spirit had a hand in there somewhere.

Friday. After spending a few weekends at St. Leo, my Friday evenings evolved into a prescribed pattern to decompress from the week's work. I occasionally would eat dinner at the clubhouse restaurant across the highway (St. Leo has a public golf course on its grounds), and then return for the brothers' evening service. Or I would drive to nearby Pancho's Villa, a

Mexican restaurant popular among the locals but a well-kept secret to the rest of the bay area. A piping hot plate of enchiladas or burritos with a couple of cold beers, topped off with a dessert of deep-fried ice cream was surely enough to help me unwind.

Saturday. My work began on Saturday. I would start the morning by praying, meditating, and focusing on a Bible story or passage that captured my attention. Monks have a fancy Latin name for letting your imagination interact with a Bible story: *lectio divina*. This is a meditative reading of Scripture rather than an intellectual study. Essentially, you select a passage or story, reflect on it as you move into a meditative or prayerful mind-set, and become attentive to what thoughts or feelings may arise. Sometimes it works for me, sometimes not.

After this, I would grab a late coffee and any leftovers remaining from the brothers' breakfast. Guests are permitted to eat breakfast, lunch, and dinner with the monks. If the weather was pleasant, I would move a chair from the back porch to the grounds overlooking the orange orchard and Lake Jovita. I called it my *hot seat*. At my side were a Bible and any other spiritual books I was reading. I was rarely sure what I wanted to accomplish for the weekend. Therefore I usually sat still to let the issues surface.

And issues did arise, generally revolving around Martha and me and our kids and the threatening cloud that our future presented. At first the issues were rumblings in my gut that took a while to sharpen into words or images I could comprehend. To help that process along, I strolled down to the water's edge, or walked around the abbey and the nearby university campus, or went into my room and ranted where no one could hear me (I hope) but God and Jesus. I didn't want other guests or the brothers to think I was nuts. Often, I had an emotional wrestling match, either with myself or with the Spirit. Is this what Jacob went through when he wrestled with an angel? I don't know. I only know that answers didn't come easily or often. To break the tension, I would go chat with a brother running the abbey's bookstore and browse through their books. I usually ate lunch with the brothers. They cracked me up with their stories—some devout, but most not.

After lunch I would return to my hot seat. In the late afternoon, I would take an hour's walk around town or head out to the country road across from the abbey. I shared the brothers' evening meal and the last service before they retired for the night. I then returned to my room to finish what was bothering me, or at least to try to put it on an emotional shelf, where both it and I could rest for the night. Sleep was sometimes restful, often fitful.

Sunday. I began as I did on Saturday—with prayer, meditation, and an attempt at *lectio divina*. Then, after checking my mood's temperature, I either would go to the brothers' morning Mass or return to my hot seat. Lunch would be my last meal with the brothers. Afterward, I packed up before having a last sit-down to reflect on the weekend and the issues that arose. Rarely were any resolved. But as I drove out from the abbey, I was often more grounded than when I drove in on Friday. I arrived home by midafternoon Sunday, ready to spend time with Martha again and to relieve the children of their caregiver duties.

PART TWO

THE PRICE OF MERCY, THE COST OF FEAR

FOUR

THE CLOSET

Don't deny the diagnosis. Try to defy the verdict.

—Norman Cousins,
Head First: The Biology of Hope

An Artful Hope

"C'mon, Carlen, we've got to get out there *now*," Martha exclaimed. *There* being the Suntan Art Center on St. Pete Beach, next door to the big pink Don Cesar hotel. Martha was displaying two of her watercolor paintings at a weekend art show. We hustled out on Friday to see them. "Look, here they are," Martha said, grabbing my hand and pulling me to the paintings. *You'd think there were no other paintings in this show,* I thought as I smiled. She beamed as she looked at them. Then she showed me their price tags: $200 each. "Judi helped me price them." Judi

Dazzio was her art teacher. We returned Sunday afternoon to see if the paintings sold. They hadn't. But that didn't matter.

Eighteen months after her diagnosis, Martha was encouraged by our sister-in-law KK to join her in an art class at the St. Petersburg Art Center. (KK Cooper is the late wife of Martha's brother Frank.) *This could get really interesting,* I thought, knowing that in our twenty-six years of marriage Martha had shown little enthusiasm for art. She loved to sing and dance and be center stage, but she wasn't into quiet hobbies such as painting or writing. Nonetheless, Martha and KK joined the watercolor painting class, which ran for three to four hours, one day a week.

Martha painted dozens of pictures large and small, including pictures of turtles and fish swimming in an orange-and-green sea, a multicolored zebra, and a blue-faced hippo walking along an orange-and-yellow rainbow. Judi would hand Martha a sketch to paint, and Martha's imagination would tap into a complexity and boldness of color not shown before.

I look at one of her paintings as I sit in our living room.[1] About two feet wide and three feet high, it hangs above the fireplace. I think it's a self-portrait, but I'm not sure that was Martha's intent. I've seen it thousands of times since we hung it more than a decade ago. I'm drawn first to the dark violet eyes with rouge-colored eyelids. They're sad, set in a strong, handsome face. From them, streams of brown tears trace paths over yellow cheeks. Her upper jaw is a swipe of pink. Her lower jaw and chin are shaded light green as they fold under to a neck swathed in brown. Her thick hair is multicolored, which would fit right in with today's edgier styles; streaks of green, brown, blue, red,

---

1   This painting can be viewed at www.carlenmaddux.com/about/.

pink, and yellow tumble down around her shoulders. Although the undercurrent of this painting is undeniable pathos, the bold colors with their odd, potent mixtures explode with joy.

Judi pulled me aside one day. "Carlen, this can't be taught," she said of Martha's use of color. "I don't know where it's coming from." As I looked at her art, I wondered, *What's going on in your mind, Martha? Why can't you be confident like this all the time?* During her spells of confidence, Martha talked clearly, remembered names and events, and realized who was present with her. *Isn't there a way to bottle this?*

The girl I married in 1972 was, if nothing else, confident. I asked her out for a first date in Atlanta. I was coaching football and teaching at a high school. Martha had moved there to teach at another high school after spending the summer as a maid at Glacier National Park. We knew each other because we both had gone to college in Atlanta. Upon arriving from Montana, Martha called me, and I drove to her apartment to help her unload the car.

"How about going out tonight?" I asked her. "I've got to scout a football game at six, so maybe we can grab something to eat after that."

"No thanks," she said, "I'm tired."

I did a double take. "Okay . . . well, then, can I come by and see you after the game?"

"Sure, that'd be great."

"I'll be back around eight-thirty," I said as I walked to my car. I got in, started it up, then turned it off and sat there for a few minutes. Finally, I walked back to Martha's apartment and knocked. "Mind if I ask you a question, Marty?" I said.

"No, what?"

"Out of curiosity, if I'd asked you to the downtown Hyatt for dinner tonight, would you have gone with me?"

"Of course," she said, grinning at me, her blue eyes dancing.

"All right," I laughed. "I just needed to know what the rules are." We married ten months later.

Sleepless in St. Petersburg

Much about alzheimer's unnerved me, but nothing more than the disappearance of Martha's confidence. Her will and initiative vanished. She often was more withdrawn than expressive, more hesitant than decisive. In hindsight, I can see that her confidence had been eroding for a while.

Eighteen months before her diagnosis, Martha decided to run for an open seat in Florida's state legislature. During the course of that primary campaign, her decision-making and actions took odd turns that I hadn't seen before in her two-decade political career. She'd been involved in over half a dozen campaigns, either as a manager or as a candidate, winning all but one. The strangest twist of this primary race came during Martha's high-profile debate with her opponent at a well-connected political group's gathering. I'd seen Martha in this kind of setting in earlier campaigns, and she'd handled them confidently. She was quick on her feet with mostly smart, practical responses. In this debate, though, she asked for questions to be repeated, and she hedged her answers. It seemed she was trying to remember a script.

As soon as we got home I asked Martha about it.

"What do you mean?" she said.

"Well," I said, and then stopped. I was surprised she didn't catch my drift. "Why weren't you able to remember the questions? And your answers seemed a bit slow and off the mark."

She looked flustered and then said, "Some guy asked me a question before we went on stage, and it confused me." But she couldn't remember the person or his question.

My gut told me that this shaky performance had cost Martha the election. And she did lose, by twenty votes.

The disappearance of Martha's confidence, more than anything else, drove me to search for a possible way out of alzheimer's beyond the bounds of medical science, which had no answer in 1997. It still doesn't. I read everything I could find on alzheimer's as well as on health in general. Some readings were mainstream, and others were way over the edge. Some were insightful; others mere bromides.

A few seemingly credible sources indicated aluminum as a possible culprit. Research suggested that by using aluminum pots and pans we were somehow leaching microscopic elements of aluminum into our food. *This is nuts,* I muttered to myself as I opened our cabinet drawers and tossed out all the aluminum cookware. A year or two later, this whole idea was debunked by more extensive research.

I even began to investigate faith healing, which cut sharply against the grain of my upbringing. Have I mentioned I was desperate? The small Tennessee town where I grew up in the 1950s saw its share of tent revivalists roll through on the sawdust trail. And several miles east, up in the Appalachians, were the snake-handling cults. These preachers also pumped up their volume on radio and TV shows. They were expert at two things—shaking fear into you and shaking money out of you.

The book *Healing* by Francis MacNutt, a former Catholic priest, was nothing like that overwrought emotionalism. The more I read, the more sense MacNutt made, and I began to take a fresh look at spiritual healing and its Christian roots. His writing directed me to his mentor, Agnes Sanford, author of a classic in the field, *The Healing Light*. She was the daughter of Presbyterian missionaries and wife of an Episcopal priest. I found Sanford's writings and approach practical and succinct.

A Reunion

That spring of 1999, when Martha was painting and I was reading these books on healing, she decided she wanted to go to her thirtieth college reunion. I was uncertain how that would turn out. Martha hadn't told any of her friends from Agnes Scott about her condition. But she was intent on showing up, so we drove to Atlanta.

At the reunion's first party, Martha and about a dozen friends got together at one of their homes. I made sure she got to the house and told her I'd be back in a couple of hours. *I hope these are good friends,* I thought as I left. Upon my return, I stepped inside where Martha was sitting and talking in a circle with other women. Two of her friends came up, walked me straight outside, and buttonholed me.

"What's the matter with Martha?" they asked.

"What did Martha tell you?" I asked them.

Not much, they said. For eighteen months, I'd tried to honor Martha's insistent wish that no one outside the family know of her diagnosis. But there was no way to avoid their questions. As I explained, the color faded from their faces. "Well, that explains it," said a friend who had a family member with dementia. I'm sure the word spread like wildfire after Martha and I drove away.

Saturday evening at the last class party it was clear to me that everyone who knew Martha knew of her diagnosis. That created an awkward response from her friends as they tried to adjust to a different Martha. Or maybe I was the one feeling awkward. As we circulated among her friends, most of them appeared comfortable with her. A few, however, were standoffish, and a couple of them fawned a bit too much over her. I let Martha make her own way among her friends, while I kept an eye on her from afar. I also kept looking around for the one person who was both Martha's friend and mine from our college years, Mary Cappleman Zahl. Finally, in she walked, and after saying hello to several friends, she came up to me and we hugged.

We exchanged a few pleasantries while trying to catch up on the last three decades, as though that were possible in fifteen minutes. Then Mary moved on to talk with her classmates, including Martha. We stayed awhile longer before Martha and I called it a night. As we worked our way out the door, I waved good-bye to Mary across the way.

On Monday my office phone rang. It was Mary Zahl. "Carlen, what's wrong with Martha?" This reunion weekend had worn that question thin. Nonetheless, after disclosing what was no longer a secret, I told her about Martha's art, what we were doing to keep her active, what the prospects were, and so on. I was unsure of Mary's take on spiritual healing, so I did a soft-shoe around my readings of Agnes Sanford and Francis MacNutt. Her response surprised me. "We had a healing conference last year at our church. I'd be happy to send you the tapes from it and a book by the speaker, if you would like."

"Who was the speaker?"

"Paul invited a friend from Australia." Mary's husband, Paul, was the minister of the Episcopal church in downtown Birmingham. He also was author of several religious books. Their friend, Canon Jim Glennon, had started a healing ministry a few decades earlier at his Anglican church in Sydney.

"I'm open to almost anything," I told Mary. *That is, anything but snake handling and folks rolling around on the floor,* I thought. Glennon's four cassette tapes and book arrived within the week.

A Look Back

I listened to the tapes after Martha went to sleep. I didn't want to bother her if I thought she wouldn't connect with them. I'd already hit enough roadblocks. I also started reading Canon Glennon's book, *Your Healing Is Within You.*

"If you've taken ill, look back six to eighteen months," Canon Glennon said on the tapes. "Look to see if there was any major stress in your life at that time." If so, it could very well be the cause of your illness, or a major contributor, he explained. I hadn't heard that before, and it hit me square on. I was aware that prolonged stress could be harmful, but not in such a two-plus-two-equals-four way. I was intrigued.

But before I went too deep, I did some investigating. That the Zahls were friends with Glennon offered a measure of comfort, as did his connection to a leading church in Australia. My comfort grew when I learned he was personal friends with the Archbishop of Canterbury and on a first-name basis with top Australian government officials. Name-dropping has no value, but I guess I needed to know that his ministry was generally well regarded and that he wasn't some fringe freelancer.

Canon Glennon makes clear that we shouldn't burden ourselves with guilt when looking back for contributing causes: *You mean I've brought this illness on myself?* The point is to resolve any emotional issues as best we can. Doing that, he says, might improve the chances of reversing the course of an illness or disease.

"I'm not saying that this approach always applies," says Glennon, "so I don't flog the issue." He emphasizes that "the healing ministry of the church seeks to work in full association with the medical profession." But he adds, "The idea of the healing ministry is not that you go to the doctor first and then say 'Amen' on the end."

"Jesus majored on the need to forgive," he says. A core theme of Jesus's teaching is that resentment cuts us off from God and can be a potent cause of illness: "If you haven't forgiven," Glennon adds, "all I can say is, 'God help you.'"

Soon Martha was listening to these tapes with me. As we did, I was reminded of Frederick Buechner's passage in his book *Wishful Thinking*: "Of the Seven Deadly Sins, anger is possibly the most fun. To lick your wounds, to smack your lips over grievances long past, to roll over your tongue the prospect of bitter confrontations still to come, to savor to the last toothsome morsel both the pain you are given and the pain you are giving back—in many ways it is a feast fit for a king. The chief drawback is that what you are wolfing down is yourself. The skeleton at the feast is you."

Click. Canon Glennon's message snapped into focus: *Unattended resentment can wreak havoc on my mind, body, and emotions.* I began to see that forgiveness is not some pious virtue that I should get around to when I'm not so busy. Instead, forgiveness, or its lack, can be a matter of life or death, of good health or ill.

Canon Glennon's fresh take—fresh for me, at least—on the potential damage that stress can cause sent me searching. I backtracked from Martha's diagnosis to sniff out any major stresses she could have endured. Several things came up on my radar: the failed campaign, the fender bender, two detached retinas, and the D&C. This was a lot, but none seemed to carry any lingering bitterness, so I continued to look.

As I scanned backward, I asked Martha about any resentment she may have, but she changed the subject. I backed off. Later I gently tried to probe a bit more. She pulled away. I backed off again. As this cycle kept repeating, I began to see a "closet" within her in which she'd stuffed the most painful things of her life. The door to that closet never opened, it seemed to me, except to stuff something else in.

I prayed and reflected on this closet. A memory arose from earlier conversations with Martha, when she was healthy. *Could that be it?* I wondered. On occasion I got into a melancholy funk, which I couldn't shake right away. "Snap out of it, Carlen," she'd say. "I'm trying to, Martha, but I can't. Give me some space." Martha had little patience with anyone's blues, especially mine. I finally piped up, "Don't you ever get down, Martha?" She quickly retorted, "I *never* get depressed." That surprised me. She was right, though. I couldn't remember her doing much in the way of self-reflection. She dealt with frustration by directing a quick temper at whoever was in her line of fire.

So that's what Martha does, I thought. *She tries to resolve a problem by getting mad and throwing it off on others. But instead, she's really shoving the pain into this closet, slamming the door shut.* I guess this was Amateur Psychology 101, but I shared this idea with a couple of close friends and a counselor, and they agreed. This image of the closet seemed to fit. It felt right.

Whenever I sniffed around this closet door, I sensed the hair on Martha's neck rising. My nose got bopped more than once. Eventually, though, Martha and I drew up a list of people we had hurt, or who had hurt us. We prayed about these relationships. We sought within our hearts to forgive and be forgiven. We asked God to shower his love on these friends and relationships—and on us. That released some deep-seated resentment within me, and it seemed to do the same for Martha.

As we recounted these hurts, one issue above all the others surfaced for Martha. About eighteen months before Martha's earliest signs of memory loss, her long-held resentment toward her father had turned white hot. Bitter about the way he continued to bully her mother verbally, Martha had insisted that her mother divorce him. Both were in their late seventies. Martha and I talked and prayed about these feelings toward her father. We asked for God's help and insight.

Meanwhile, our eighteen-year-old Kathryn also heard Canon Glennon's comments on forgiveness. One day she turned to Martha and said, "Mommie, isn't it time you forgive Granddaddy?"

Martha looked at Kathryn, then at me. "Yes," she said in a matter-of-fact way. My jaw went slack. Kathryn's simple question had cracked open four decades of hoarded bitterness. I thought, *"Out of the mouth of babes . . ."* *they say.* As we prayed, Martha spoke three words I'd never heard from her: "I forgive Daddy." We all cried.

"What do you want to do?" I asked Martha. "Do you want to tell him? Or write him? Or do nothing right now?"

"I want to write him," she said. "Can you help?"

"Why don't you dictate to me what you want to say?" I offered. "Then you can copy that in your own handwriting." This is the note Martha wrote:

> *May 20, 1999*
> *Dear Dad,*
> *For many years I did not want to be around you because of your anger. It seems now, though, that your anger has subdued. So I feel better, and I want to love you again.*
> *I hope this letter does not hurt our relationship. I need to know that you forgive me for holding these feelings for so long while I forgive you for your anger.*
> *I do love you and hope you love me too. I've prayed to God to forgive both you and me.*
> *Love, Marty*

When she dropped the note in the mailbox the next day, it looked as though a fog of anxiety and bitterness had lifted, and Martha broke into a genuine smile, one that I hadn't seen in a long time. We celebrated by going out for dinner that night.

The impact of these events stirred something within me for weeks. I mulled over Martha's closet and her relief in forgiving her father, about resentment's potential for destruction, and about Kathryn's serendipitous question. I grew acutely aware that I'd been so focused on Martha that I hadn't realized that I also had a closet full of dull pain within me. I too had opened that door only to shove more hurt inside, never to be aired out. It finally dawned on me: *I need to be healed in my own way as much as Martha does in hers.*

FIVE

ELVIS, DAD, JESUS, AND ME

Light breaks where no sun shines.

—title of Dylan Thomas poem

Martha and I grabbed a seat halfway back in the sanctuary. A ragtag band led a couple hundred of us in singing; then the minister rose to speak. As he talked, I was thinking: *I sure hope something good comes out of this. Martha needs to get well soon. I don't know how long I can keep up this caregiving.* It had been two years since she was diagnosed with alzheimer's.

I was wary of traveling the hundred miles to this two-day healing conference in Winter Park. Martha hadn't done well at a similar event a year earlier. So while I wanted to learn as much as I could, I also wanted to make sure Martha was comfortable.

The guest speaker was Canon Jim Glennon's successor at the healing ministry in Australia, Canon Jim Holbeck. Like Glennon, Holbeck spoke about our need to forgive if we want to experience healing. I asked myself, *Does Martha have other resentments that she hasn't faced? Is any bitterness still lingering after forgiving her father?*

I was so focused on Martha that I didn't see the curve ball hurtling my way when Canon Holbeck delivered these words: "Our feelings for our earthly father often shape our feelings for our heavenly Father." It hit me square between the eyes, setting loose a series of questions about God's love that had been bothering me since Martha's diagnosis. Whenever I had tried to understand my relationship with God, I'd drawn a blank. But that night, one question flowed into the next like dominoes.

Isn't it my duty to love God?

Jesus told us: "You shall love the Lord your God with all your heart, and with all your soul, and with all your strength, and with all your mind" (Mk. 12:30). *Okay then, why don't I?*

Isn't God supposed to love me? I'd heard all my life that he does, but I'd rarely felt any love from him.

Is my relationship with Dad the reason I don't feel God's love—or feel any love for God?

These kept turning over in my mind: *Did Dad love me? Does God? Do I love Dad? God?*

Man in Charge

Dad carried a key ring with what seemed like fifty keys to my young eyes. Keys to our house, keys to his store, keys to the church, and keys to whatever else he had charge over. Dad owned a hardware store in our small country town in Tennessee. Maddux Hardware must have housed a jillion different items—big things such as wood-burning stoves and plows, and little things such as two-penny nails and seed corn. And he knew where every last item was, or where it should have been. Dad was the man in charge.

Dad also was a man in charge at the church he helped start, serving as an elder for almost four decades. My brother, my sister, and I knew our duty there too. We were to go religiously to three services a week—Sunday morning, Sunday evening, and Wednesday evening. I'm certain Dad and Mom wanted us to learn about God and Jesus. But I also suspect that as one of three or four long-standing elders, Dad wanted our family to be seen as a model in this small church in a town where you knew nearly everyone.

As a young kid, I knew I was supposed to get baptized around the seventh or eighth grade. The church I grew up in called that period in our lives the "age of accountability." That's when I'd be held accountable by God for my thoughts and actions. And I didn't look forward to it. Before reaching that age I'd been thinking, *I can get away with pretty much anything . . . within reason, of course. God won't hold it against me. But once I become "accountable," watch out! Everything will change. God will start taking notes, and he'll hold on to them for the rest of my life.* To this kid's eyes, baptism was a major step in convincing God to tear up a lot of those notes when my "day of judgment" came. Or so I hoped.

Our church's baptisms were not a weak-tea variety that involves sprinkling or pouring water. Ours was a full dunking in a tank big enough to be an extra-large hot tub. The day I decided to get baptized, the preacher "made a call" for anyone who felt moved to come forward. I took a deep breath and walked up to the front of the church, shaking inside.

"Do you repent and confess your sins to God, Carlen?" the preacher asked as I stood there.

"Yes, I do," I whispered in front of Mom and Dad and my brother and sister and Grandmother and Grandpa and all the congregation, not to mention God and Jesus and my buddies in the back row of the balcony, smirking. Scores of eyes were bearing down on the back of my neck.

I then walked through a door at the front of the sanctuary, accompanied by the preacher and another man who helped me get ready for the baptism. I put on a robe after stripping off all my Sunday go-to-meeting clothes. I could hear the congregation's muffled singing in the background, voices only since our church didn't believe in the use of musical instruments.

"Are you ready, Carlen?" the preacher asked.

"Yes, sir," I responded, my voice quivering.

The preacher and I walked out from the room, through a hallway, and down the steps into the baptismal tank at the front of the sanctuary. As I stood chest-deep in the water, the curtains to the baptismal were drawn back so the congregation could witness this event. The singing hushed. The preacher held his right arm upward, said a few words, and then lowered me backward into the water as I squeezed my nose. It seemed as if I was held under for a long while, but he lifted me back up just in time for me to catch my breath. Water streamed off my flattop onto my peach-fuzzed face.

After the service, church members came up to congratulate me, and my mom and dad and grandparents all said how glad they were that I'd made this decision. "I'm proud of you, Carlen," Dad said as he shook my hand. And that was that. No hugs or kisses, just a handshake and a congratulatory word or two from Dad. *What just happened?* I wondered after I got home. A year or two earlier, Dad had given me his brief-and-to-the-point "sex talk." Brief though that was, it was more than any discussion we had about my baptism. As an adult today, I wonder: *If being baptized was that important, why didn't Dad talk with me about it? And where was the emotional warmth that could have driven home its significance?*

Dad seemed to enjoy being in charge at church and at work. But as a young adult, he wanted most to be in charge in the US Navy. He'd wanted to be an admiral. Although I never heard Dad or anyone else in the family say that, I could feel it and see it. The dress sword and scabbard he received when graduating from the Naval Academy hung in a prominent place above the entrance to our living room. His full dress uniform hung in a closet. And his Navy dress hat sat on a shelf where I could pull it down, plop it on my head, and march around the house. Dad had gone to college in our hometown for three years before spending another four at Annapolis. He was unable to pull combat duty in World War II because of a back injury. Instead, he held down a desk job. He resigned after the war.

In some ways, my brother, sister, and I became that naval unit Dad didn't get to command. Each school day, Dad woke us at 6:45 AM sharp. On his first round through he flipped on our lights, and from my bedroom door said, "Rise 'n' shine, Carlen. I want to see your feet on the floor when I come back." When he came back through I was still lying in bed, but my feet dangled off the side, toes touching the floor. "Okay, Carlen, straighten up." And I did. I don't remember him coming into the room, sitting on the bed, waking me with a back scratch or a kiss or a hug. It was not quite *The Sound of Music*'s von Trapp family, but Dad indeed was the captain of our family ship while Mom played the Julie Andrews role with us kids.

Distant as Dad could be, he wasn't abusive to us, either physically or verbally. He took good care of us. During summers, my brother and I worked at his store in the mornings to earn our allowance, and then he let us off to play tennis. We took summer trips as a family through nearly all forty-eight contiguous states. He made sure we had activities to do year-round—football, baseball, basketball, golf, swimming, and tennis—and encouraged us to do our best in all we did. I earned two of the Boy Scouts' highest awards—Eagle Scout and God & Country—made straight A's in high school, was the quarterback on our football team, and started at center on our basketball team.

In the spring of 1963 I agreed to attend Georgia Tech on a full football scholarship. I was both pumped and overwhelmed as I thought about leaving my hometown, population eight thousand, to go to college in a big city like Atlanta. Yet Dad's response to the most important decision I'd made in my seventeen years was pretty matter-of-fact. "I was hoping you'd do that," Dad said. "Bobby Dodd was my football hero in high school." Dodd was Georgia Tech's head coach. Beyond that, our conversation focused more on perfunctory matters than on any excitement Dad may have had for what I'd accomplished. Maybe I wanted too much from

Dad—maybe more than any father of that generation was capable of giving in a time when men often were expected to do their duty yet not display any affection. Still, a full-body hug and a big wide grin would have been nice—some emotional exclamation point that said, "This is my boy—isn't he something!"

Our feelings for our earthly father often shape our feelings for our heavenly Father.

My dad was a good man. Dad was a responsible man. Dad was a man in charge. Yet as my father, he was an emotionally distant man. And that's how I imagined my heavenly Father: *God is good. God is in charge. God is distant.*

I'm All Shook Up

A few days after that healing conference in Winter Park, I was trying to meditate in our living room before Martha awoke. As I did, I reflected again on Dad and God and me and our so-called love. A tranquil silence settled over me that October morning, a stillness that seemed to come from a presence beyond me.

OCTOBER 13, 1999

As I sat on our couch, my mind swept back to my frustration of not feeling God's love. I could conceptualize that love to an extent, I could believe it's there, but I'd rarely felt it in my bones. Adding to this frustration was the sense that I was blocking the flow of God's healing Spirit over Martha. My efforts were all about striving, with no resting in the Spirit.

As I puzzled over this, my mind and heart flashed back to an incident four decades earlier that I'd forgotten. I was ten or eleven. Elvis was coming on the scene, and I'd been practicing his moves with an air guitar in my bedroom, behind a locked door. I pouted and tried to make my eyes look sultry, all while swiveling my hips and knees to "All Shook Up" and "You Ain't Nothin' but a Hound Dog."

After I had Elvis's moves down—as good as any kid one step from puberty could—I decided to try them out on Dad. We were standing in our front hallway with its floor-to-ceiling mirror when I jumped in front of him, saying, "Hey Dad, look at this." I started to sing "Hound Dog" but got no further than two strums on my air guitar and one swivel of the hips before Dad cut me off. "I never want to see you do that again. Do you understand? Go on, get out of here!"

I tucked tail and ran up to my room. I understood that I did something wrong, but I didn't understand what. What's this I'm feeling? Guilt? Why? What'd I do? I kept asking as I withdrew further into myself.

Forty years later, these questions prompted strong emotions within me. I saw something I hadn't realized before: With that incident my heart and mind had begun to separate from each other. I no longer wanted to reveal my feelings to Dad. I could talk ideas with him but not feelings. I thought I'd be reprimanded if I revealed to him my doubts and fears about God or about playing football, or my questions about girls and sex. I decided the "manly" thing to do was to buck up and keep those things hidden.

While still meditating in our living room, I puzzled over this four-decade-old memory: What am I supposed to do with this? Instantly, I felt a tug on the sleeve of my imagination. It was not something I prompted. It was a coaxing from deep within. This tug brought me face-to-face with Dad.

In my mind's eye, Jesus had one arm around Dad's shoulders and the other draped over mine.

I felt impelled to ask Dad, "Why did you cut me off when I showed you my Elvis moves?"

Jesus turned to Dad: "Do you understand, Dave, what you did to Carlen?"

"No, I didn't then. But I do now."

Dad turned to me. "Carlen, I was wrong." He began to cry. "I would give anything if I could take it back. I can't, but I'm asking you now to forgive me, if you can." He went on to say that his authoritarian attitude in raising us had been misguided in many ways.

Then Jesus looked directly into my eyes, saying not a word. His penetrating look startled me, but I knew the question he was not asking.

"Yes, Dad, I do forgive you," I said with no further prompting. "And I need you to forgive me for being so secretive with you, for not sharing my thoughts and feelings."

"Of course I do, Carlen. I love you," he said, his eyes still moist.

Hearing these words, in the midst of this deep meditation, my heart flooded with joy and tears. I shook and cried until there were no more tears to shed. As the intensity of this emotion subsided, Mom and my sister, Alice, and brother, Bob, appeared in this scene. All five of us talked up a storm. We laughed our hearts out, as we might say in the South. Dad was anything but distant. Nor did I sense any hint of the cat-and-mouse game I'd played with Dad for years, that game of not wanting him to know my feelings about almost anything.

All this began to fade from my imagination when I heard Dad call out, "Hey, Carlen, look at this." And he began to swivel like Elvis—hips, knees, pouting lips, air guitar, and all. Then in my mind's eye we all started laughing and rockin' and rollin', playing our guitars, and singing "Hound Dog." Even Mom and Jesus. With that, the whole scene passed from my view, our laughter fading.

I was spent. Sitting there that October morning on the couch in our living room, I was engulfed in a deep love for Dad that I'd never felt. And what must have been our heavenly Father's love seeped into my heart, mind, and body, warming all. I am loved, I thought. And I love.

At long last my heart and mind were melting into one. Out of this calm I whispered aloud, "Thank you, my Father. Thank you, my Master Jesus. Thank you, my Spirit, for loving my family and me so. Amen."

As this encounter drew to a close, I didn't know whether this was a passing emotion or something that would precipitate a significant change within me. Since then, I've seen God's love appear in many sizes, shapes, shades, and forms. For instance, when our children were young, Martha and I would take them to the beach for a week in the summer. In my moments alone, I'd lie flat on my back at the water's edge, soaking up the setting sun, letting the Gulf waves flow over me and back out. That's how I've recently felt God's love on occasion—flowing into me and back out, into me and out, in and out. As it has flowed inward, my God's tender, healing touch has caressed my heart. And as it has ebbed, I have felt the poisons in my mind being drawn out—poisons of bitterness, self-righteousness, and cynicism.

I've also continued to think a lot about Dad in recent years. Only twice do I remember him opening his heart to me. When Mom died in 1974, Dad was hurting, and he appeared lost. And then, when he lay at death's door two decades later, he held both my hands as he told me, "I love you, Carlen." My feelings for Dad softened both times as his heart cracked open, but I didn't know what to do in either case other than to grieve for him—and for Bob, Alice, and me.

I now see the good in Dad that I hadn't seen before this meditation on the Elvis memory. One trait stands out above all the others—his laugh. Dad's was a full-bodied laugh with no hint of cynicism. In the mid-1950s, Santa Claus gave our family a Christmas-gift trip to Florida. Mom and Dad slept on the double bed in an economy motel, and we three kids were on the floor in sleeping bags. When it was my turn to shower, I saw several sets of disposable paper slippers, which I thought—perfectly logically—were to be worn while taking a shower. After all, they were labeled "shower shoes." *Wow, these are really nice,* I thought. *I've never seen these before.* Not long into my shower, with paper slippers snug on my feet, I called out to the family, "These shoes can really get soggy." Dad was the first to burst out laughing. Mom, Bob, and Alice quickly chimed in. I was clueless as to why that was funny. After catching his breath, Dad explained to me the intricate mechanics of disposable shower shoes.

My love for Dad continues to flow ever more fully now even though he's been gone for more than two decades. Had I not meditated in this way on this Elvis memory, the odds are great that my feelings for Dad would still be obscure and hardened. And in all likelihood I would still be asking my God: *Where's your warmth? Where's your help? Where's your love?*

SIX

ALONE IN THOMAS MERTON'S CABIN

The devil of resentment is that it's so often justified.
But who do you think pays the piper?

—Canon Jim Glennon

I drove out that Sunday in July thinking, *I sure hope this week will be worth it.* This would be the longest time I'd been away from Martha since she was diagnosed with alzheimer's four years earlier. I was going on a personal retreat at the Abbey of Gethsemani, the monastery we had visited in Kentucky. Martha could take care of herself but in a limited capacity, so I couldn't leave her alone. Her mother and our sister-in-law KK would be watching after her at our summer cabin in Montreat, North Carolina.

"Montreat's my home," Martha often told me. As a child and as an adult, she spent her summers there, forming lifelong friendships. And she made sure our children did too. Before Martha considered marrying me, I had to pass a few tests. Not only did I have to love her and her pup Collie-Cocoa, I also had to love Montreat. And . . . I do. Montreat is a Presbyterian conference center set within a town of the same name. The town is situated in a cove surrounded on three sides by mountains; there's only one way in and out. Montreat is one of those rare places where you don't think twice about leaving your house unlocked.

That Sunday, after lunch, I hugged Martha and kissed her good-bye as we stood on the front porch. "I'll see you Saturday," I said, letting her hands slip from mine. Martha stood beside her mother waving while I pulled out of the driveway. As I drove out through the entrance gate with the letters *M-O-N-T-R-E-A-T* embedded in its brown limestone arch, I had a vague twilight-zone sense that I was slipping from an old, familiar world into a new, uncharted one.

I headed west over the Smokies, then turned north into Kentucky. Six hours later, I pulled into Gethsemani just as the sun dropped behind the hills, or knobs, above me. I checked in with the brother in charge, and he directed me to a cabin a mile from the abbey community. Other guests were staying in a four-story retreat center near the church. When I'd called a few months earlier to reserve space, a brother had said, "Since the retreat center is filled, would you be okay staying in Thomas Merton's hermitage?" I answered, "Sure, that's fine," trying to remain casual about such a prospect. I admire Merton for his wit and prolific writing, and also for his willingness to swim against current conventions—religious and political. Yet for me, the singular trait of this complex man is his simple humility. Merton lived his last years in this cabin, seeking even greater solitude, away from the abbey and its activities.

Arriving at the cabin, I was struck by its setting at the top of a knoll with woods to the left, right, and rear and a clearing to the front. A range of knobs outlined the distant horizon to the east. As dusk covered the scene, I saw deer dart across the clearing, some stopping to gather around the salt lick fifty yards out. Later that evening, after listening to a homily by Martha's friend and mine Fr. Matthew Kelty, two rabbits greeted me while I was walking along the gravel road leading back to the cabin. By week's end the deer and rabbits and I became, if not good friends, familiar faces.

I went to Gethsemani for two reasons: first, to catch a break from the day-to-day grind of having to cope with Martha's declining abilities; and second, to seek a clearer understanding of what was going on within her. My exploration of spiritual healing led me to think that Martha's condition could have been provoked as much by issues of emotional distress as by physiological ones. I went to seek guidance and understanding by which to address these issues. Gethsemani is marked by its commitment to silence, prayer, and hospitality. And within the solitude of its woods, I was able to relax, read, pray, think, wrestle with God, and most importantly, rest in him.

My daily routine was pretty simple: Wake up at six o'clock. Go sit on the front porch and open the day with prayer and meditation while reflecting on stories from Mark's Gospel. Get dressed and eat breakfast before going to work. By work, I mean calling on the Spirit to open me up, to help me understand

Martha's feelings; and to wait, give thanks, and listen. I also tried to reflect on Jesus's death, his resurrection, his ascension, his relationships, and his teachings. I sought to remind myself that his mind was transforming my mind, and his heart, my heart.

During my first three days at Gethsemani, I broke no new ground in understanding the cause of Martha's condition. When no connection came, I read books that challenged my thinking and beliefs. Or I walked around the clearing out front. Then I turned back to the Spirit, seeking to allow her warm, healing light to bathe my heart, mind, and body.

On the morning of my fourth day, Wednesday, I again asked God's Spirit to offer me insight into Martha's feelings, to put me in her shoes, to let me know her fears, to let me see and hear the way she sees and hears. Again, that didn't happen. Instead, my attention was drawn to my family, to my childhood and teen years. I'd already reconciled much with my father. Yet more work apparently needed to be done. As I pictured Dad and Mom, I grew angry with them for raising me in the church they did. Its fundamentalist teachings, untouched by grace, imposed a needless restraint on this little boy who just wanted to please his parents. Next I got mad at Dad's parents, members of the same church. Then I yelled at God for allowing me to grow up in such a suffocating setting.

These tirades dissolved into silent reflection. And soon, an awareness of two ugly character traits I possessed arose from the depths of my heart. *You're not exactly perfect yourself, Carlen*, they announced. An unseemly smugness and a frosty self-righteousness have beset me my whole life. Too often they have kept me shackled to a cold, dark wall of fear. In the worst of days, my life has felt gray, hopeless, and not much worth living. I sensed those two traits bubbling within as I sat on the grassy clearing in front of the cabin, corroding my insides until I could do nothing but cry out, *Help me, God! Free me—I want to be freed from this ugliness. Please . . . help me.*

I saw nothing, and I heard nothing.

Where's God when I need him? I asked. As soon as I said *need him,* my attention shifted from my self-indulgence back to my family. A truth hammered on my heart: *Now's the time,* it pounded, *to reconcile with your family. Completely.*

Why now? I asked. *My parents aren't alive.* Mom had died years earlier at age fifty-six; Dad, at seventy-seven. Then I flashed back to my encounter with Elvis, Dad, and Jesus. I was reminded that Christ's Spirit transcends time, space, and death. Odd thoughts began to drift up: *If you want to be freed of your ugly ways, Carlen, then forgive. If you want to be released from this fear, then let go of your bitter grasping.*

Jesus, I said, *I'm trying to be as honest as I can. But I'm not sure I know how to release feelings I've held this long inside me. I need help.* I continued to pray for insight. Then as best I could, I forgave Mom and Dad. I did the same with my father's parents. And I even made peace with their church. Finally, heaven forbid, I forgave God himself. I turned to all of them in my heart and asked, *Can you still accept me despite these deep resentments?*

After a long spell, I sensed that they did, God included.

And with the certainty of this shared mercy, I felt the cold iron of fear and self-absorption snap loose from my neck and wrists. My heart leapt with joy. For reasons unclear to me, I began to say my full name aloud: *David Carlen Maddux.* As I pronounced

David—my father's name too—my breath caught and my eyes welled as I voiced these words for the first time in my life: *Yes, Dad . . . I am . . . I'm . . . Dad, I'm honored to carry your name.* I wailed loudly in the solitude of those woods during that hour of mercy. For the next forty-eight hours, I saw myself, my family, and my world through dew-tipped eyes. My step had a lift, and my spirit a lilt. I felt the ground of my heart shifting.

A Letter from Gethsemani

Friday was my last day at Gethsemani. I hoped I could get a clearer insight into Martha's condition before I left, but I had no assurance of that happening. After waking up, I sat on the front porch to meditate and pray. A couple of deer crossed the clearing out front on the way to their day's activities. I went back inside for breakfast. As I ate, I again glanced around Merton's spare cabin to mark it in my memory. From my seat in the little kitchen, I could see most of the cabin's interior with its concrete block walls. To my left was Merton's bedroom, where I slept on the only cot. To the other side was a small prayer room with a kneeling altar facing a simple wooden icon of Jesus on the cross. In front of me was the living room, dominated by a rough-hewn stone fireplace. A small bookshelf stood in the far corner with a rocking chair nearby. Next to it, a large wooden writing table spread beneath three windows, through which I could see the distant horizon. I presumed the cabin was arranged much like Merton had left it thirty-three years earlier, when he died in an accident in Bangkok. Later, I realized that Merton, who was born the same year as Dad, was at the time of his death only a year older than I when Martha was diagnosed with alzheimer's. I was fifty-two then. Not that this meant anything, other than I found comfort in this correlation with a man I respect, whose writings opened my eyes to the possibility of an intimate God.

After breakfast, I returned to the front porch, which was a simple slab of concrete with a roof overhead. Once again I asked the Spirit for help in understanding any distress that might be afflicting Martha. Nothing happened. Shortly, I sensed a stirring within my heart. The events that subsequently transpired were important enough that I wrote a letter in my journal to Martha and her parents upon my return home. But I never shared it with her parents, who have since died.

So why do I share it now, years after its writing? For one, the events I describe have served as a compass, helping me recalibrate my spiritual bearings. And these events rewired my relationship with Martha, with her parents, with each of our children, and with my sense of self. I suspect many families are not unlike Martha's and mine—we're not the only ones beset with dysfunctional behavior. The Bible, in fact, is ripe with stories of dysfunctional families. Even Jesus on occasion rudely put down his mother, father, and siblings. Some friends might not recognize Martha's parents in my letter, but I trust it's understood that I'm not sharing this merely to, as they say, air dirty laundry.

If I've learned anything from Canon Jim Glennon, it is this: Carrying spite and resentment—no matter how right I am or how much I've been wronged—can wreak havoc on my mind and body. These matters must be resolved if healing is to have a chance of unfolding.

JULY 2001

To my dear Martha and to Grace Elizabeth and Frank,

I'm writing you about my stay at Gethsemani because the most significant event of this week involves each of you. What I'm sharing I saw and heard and felt in that chamber of my heart where the Spirit invited me to dance. The Spirit's touch was light, her voice gentle, and her step firm. This was a dance of love, and I was willing to join in.

I asked the Spirit to invite me into Martha's heart, to be granted insight into her condition. Instead, the Spirit turned my attention to her parents. Looking at them, a bitterness boiled up in my heart while I recounted the stories I'd heard from Martha about her childhood: the almost daily rage and verbal abuse by Frank; the children scattering to their rooms; their mother withdrawing to her sewing room; and the pressure by Grace Elizabeth to make Martha into someone she didn't want to be.

I raged at God: "And what effect did this have on Martha's condition?"

There was no answer.

Then I heard a voice that could only have been Christ Jesus's: "Carlen, are you going to forgive Martha's parents?"

I fidgeted. I turned away. I had no good answer to this question. I could see no good qualities. "No," I finally told Jesus. "I can't. And I won't." He asked me again, his eyes reminding me of all the mercy and grace he'd granted me. I didn't say a word but got up from my chair and walked *a hundred yards out in front of the cabin and back, all the while saying, "I'm trying to, but I can't."*

Jesus eyed me, then turned to Martha's mother. "Grace Elizabeth, you worked hard to feed and dress your children and run the house. You brought them up the best you could. But what they needed most—the nurture and care of their feelings and dreams, a touch at the right moment, a hug—you didn't know how to give, did you? Can you see the toll it's taken on Martha and her brothers? And on you?

"Your lack of nurture and Frank's abusive rages rendered your family emotionally barren. Martha's plight is but a manifestation of this. Only grace and mercy by each of you can break this scourge. Can't you see, Grace Elizabeth?"

She looked stunned. Finally she murmured, "Yes." Tears streaming, she continued: "Yes I do. I'd give anything to go back and hold Martha when she wanted to cry, to pick up all my children and laugh with them."

Jesus turned and asked Martha whether she forgave her mother. A long pause. Martha through tears said yes, she did. "And I ask you, Mom, to forgive me for the harsh, rude, and angry ways I've treated you."

Grace Elizabeth put her arms around Martha. "My sweet girl, of course I do." Both cried and hugged.

"Now, Martha, can you forgive your father?"

Martha didn't blink. "No."

Jesus abruptly turned his back to us and looked straight at Frank. "Your charm with people outside your family is remarkable, Frank. You worked hard to provide for your family. But you took the gift of work and turned it into an obsession. When you came home in the evenings your bile flowed over your family, shriveling everyone's heart. Your wife and children would have loved to enjoy your warmth and charm. The good you've done is all but lost."

The blood drained from Frank's face. Averting his eyes, he said in a pained, halting voice, "Yes . . . yes I see that now. And it hurts me to know that I hurt the people I love most."

"Why don't you and Martha talk to each other?"

"Marty, I'm sorry I hurt you," Frank said with tears streaming. "But I didn't know any other way. That's the way my father treated me. Can you forgive me?"

Martha gazed at her father with cold eyes. "I will on one condition."

"What's that?"

"Tell Mom what you've told me and apologize to her."

Frank balked. I sensed an ugly pride rearing up. Jesus grabbed Frank by both shoulders and whispered to him. Within seconds, Frank turned to his wife and said with a grace I'd never heard from him, "Honey Babe, I've done wrong. I wish I could redo the past sixty years, but all I can do is tell you I'm sorry to have hurt you so. I do love you."

The tension within Grace Elizabeth melted. She looked twenty years younger. "I've wanted to hear those words our whole marriage, Frank. All I wanted was to be loved. I'm truly sorry for being so spiteful to you." They hugged, dissolving what appeared to be decades of grief.

"Now, Martha, are you ready to forgive your father?"

"Yes, I am," she cried. "You've caused a lot of pain and hurt, Daddy, but I do forgive you now."

Frank's body shook as they embraced. "Marty, you've always been the apple of my eye." Lifelong issues melted from Martha's face.

"It's time, Carlen," Jesus said. "Can you forgive Grace Elizabeth and Frank?"

I looked at Martha, then at her parents. "Yes, I can now. And I apologize to you both for the bitterness I've felt toward you."

With that, the Spirit drew this dance to a close, the release of long-hidden abuses and resentments now complete.

Christ Jesus closed this powerful, sacred dance with these words: "As you've forgiven each other, I forgive you. Care for one another. Be gentle and love each other as I love you."

With these words echoing in my heart, I close this letter. I love you dearly, Martha, and your parents.

Carlen

These intense two hours left me crying for rest. Yet joy and thanksgiving overflowed within. *What's taken place here needs to be affirmed,* I thought. I walked up to the abbey office to see if I could find Fr. Matthew. The qualities and quirks blended in this aging monk make for a curious yet wonderful Irish brew. However, one trait stands above all. For that I call him the Monk of Mercy.

He was in his office, and I shared this afternoon encounter with him. He told me, "If you don't forgive, the cycle can repeat itself from one generation to the next. God needs a channel through which to work his mercy and healing. Thanks go to our God for using you. We have no idea how God will work from this point forward. The important thing is that a channel is open for him. All you must do now is wait and watch and listen." He then lifted a prayer of blessing and mercy.

Last Dance

Exhausted, I returned to Merton's cabin at four-thirty in the afternoon and made notes on what I'd seen and heard within my heart. After resting, I stepped outside into the cool dark night. My heart skipped more than a beat at the sight above—a vast orchestration of stars. All week, no star had broken through the clouded sky. But on this silent night, unblemished by artificial light, I saw and heard a distant orchestra from deep within the constellations above. It was accompanying my Creator and his angels as they sang with one voice the primeval "Hallelujah" chorus—for Martha, for our children, for her parents, for our families, and for me. I lay on the warm ground, speechless, my spirit magnified.

This is like the night you were born, isn't it, Jesus? I exclaimed. *Martha and I thank you with naked, newborn hearts.* After a couple of hours, I stepped back into the cabin and climbed into bed, letting sleep pull its covers over me.

The next morning I went outside to bid my deer good-bye, but they were nowhere in sight. *How disappointing,* I thought, my shoulders slumping. Then I glanced above and saw two magnificent hawks turning, soaring, arcing, as if performing a silent prayer. *How appropriate for this last hour,* I thought, *this winged kiss of silence.* I closed the door to Thomas Merton's hermitage and drove out the entrance of the monastery, its cross standing high on the knob above.

SEVEN

18,000 MILES TO SYDNEY AND OTHER DAY TRIPS

But seek first [God's] kingdom and his righteousness,
and all these things shall be yours as well.

—Jesus, Matthew 6:33

June 2002. Two days before our thirtieth wedding anniversary, I was fixing breakfast when I heard a *thud!* in our bedroom. I dashed up the steps to find Martha lying on the floor, her body shaking and cramping, her expression reminiscent of that painting "The Scream." *This must be a seizure.* I'd heard about them but hadn't seen one. *What should I do?* I was too frightened to move. But something pushed me, and I remembered to make sure that Martha was far enough from our bed, the wall, or anything else that she might hit. *Check her mouth. Check her tongue. Find something to let her bite down on.* Where these thoughts came from I don't know. Maybe from my Boy Scout days.

As suddenly as the seizure began, it stopped. And Martha fell into a deep sleep on the floor. I couldn't wake her, so I lifted her onto our bed to rest. Then I called 911. The paramedics arrived, siren blaring, and swept both Martha and me off to the emergency room. While the attendants monitored Martha, I called our children and Martha's parents. The family soon gathered in the ER around Martha's bed, none of us sure of what to do but wring our hands. All the while, Martha slept.

The doctors moved Martha into the hospital to observe her for a few days. That would have been all right, but the nurses clearly had not worked with someone in Martha's condition—incontinent, disoriented, unable to talk or feed herself. She was five years into this alzheimer's. All the nurses knew to do was sedate her, per the doctor's orders, and keep her in a semiconscious state. The hospital stay was awful for the staff, judging by the impatience displayed by a few nurses. It was awful for us too.

This three-day ordeal wore me out. But I was even more exhausted from a relentless onslaught of fear. The image of Martha's body and face being wrenched by this full seizure kept scrolling through my mind. I had no forewarning that alzheimer's might precipitate a seizure, and I feared what it might portend.

When Martha came home, she was lost in a daze, much more so than previously. I didn't know if that was caused by the seizure itself or by the meds used to sedate her. Regardless, I swore that if Martha had another seizure we were not returning to the hospital. How would I handle a seizure at home? I had no idea. But I wanted to figure it out if possible. And I wanted to understand how not to give in to these fears, how not to yield to their compulsive churning.

Pointing the Bone

Reflecting on this seizure and its aftermath, I remembered listening to a tape of Canon Jim Glennon about three years earlier. I heard him describe a long-standing practice among Australia's Aboriginal tribes. If a man breaks a taboo, the witchdoctor may come to him, pull the leg bone of a bird from a bag, and point it at the man. "Pointing the bone," says Canon Glennon, "means that because the man has broken a tribal taboo, he is going to die. There are documented cases of him falling down dead at once. He will almost certainly die within a few days because he believes he's going to die."

I asked myself, *Is this for real?* An Internet search seems to verify this practice and that its consequences are, or were, real.

So what is the point? Glennon continues: "We all have faith, and if you believe that you've got a disease that's fatal, that's your faith. You believe you're going to die. And in our culture, a disease like cancer goes around like a roaring lion, seeking whom it will devour (paraphrase of 1 Pet. 5:8). It's hard to draw on healing in those circumstances because the bone has been pointed—and you accepted it."

When I first heard this, I shrank from the thought that Martha, our children, and I had been branded. A dread burned deep within me—the bone of alzheimer's was pointed at us, and I had accepted its consequences. *How can we get rid of this?* If ever I was going to think and see clearly, I knew I must shake this fear of being so branded, and if I could, maybe it would help Martha too.

I need to talk to Canon Glennon. I called Mary Zahl and asked if she could introduce us. "I should be able to. Give me a few days." Mary called back. "Canon Glennon says he would be happy to talk with you." I faxed him a note, introducing myself and telling him why I wanted to talk with him. We set a telephone date for two weeks later.

My nerves were all a-jitter. "I know you're busy, Canon Glennon. I'll be as brief as I can."

"I have ample time, Carlen," he said, putting me at ease.

"I'm enjoying your tapes and book. They're starting to make sense to me. But I've got to tell you, Canon Glennon: I'm scared. Really scared. And I don't know how to shake this fear of alzheimer's."

"We all get scared; that's not the issue," he said. "The issue is what we do with the fear. Or, what we let the fear do to us." He reminded me that it was his nervous breakdown early in his pastoral career that began his search for ways that God heals.

"It's most important that we understand what God has provided for us. Many Christians have heard that Jesus took our sins to the cross when he died, but very few realize that he also took our sickness and infirmity. Don't take my word for it," Cannon Glennon told me. "Study the Bible until you're confident of God's healing presence today."

"I've learned to cast my burden on the Lord, and I don't take it back. I reckon it has died with Christ, and I'm dead to it," he said. "That's theology. Well . . . that's *my* theology."

I'd heard enough for the time being, and I thanked him for the call. "One last thing," he added. "If you're going to have faith, don't pray about the problem. You'll never get healed that way. We need to understand where we're heading, Carlen. Am I moving toward the fulfillment of my fears and problems? Or toward the acceptance of God's kingdom, perfect and complete in every respect?"

"I understand, I think." Jim's comments—he asked me to call him Jim—energized me, yet I was confused.

Don't Look Back

After a few sleepless nights, I decided to shift my focus away from the symptoms afflicting Martha. *That sounds fairly simple and might be the easiest thing to do for now,* I thought. Jim suggested physically turning around 180 degrees whenever I was overcome by fear. And then repeating something like this: "I turn away from these symptoms, and as I do I turn unto God's face and depend on him more."

Turning physically was the easy part. Letting go of these fears was not. I hadn't anticipated having to make a dozen turns or more every hour. It made me dizzy. I was disheartened by Martha's loss of confidence and ability to talk. All I could see in my mind was her slowly shrinking away toward death—and the unraveling of our family. I knew fear was powerful, but I had not realized how much it could mesmerize me.

I kept plugging away, yet with little progress. An ancient biblical story recounts how Lot's wife turned into a "pillar of salt" after looking back on the destruction of Sodom and Gomorrah. I felt the truth of that story in my bones. The more I tried to turn toward God's face, the more fear's tentacles drew me back.

I felt my heart and mind turning into a block of salt, for I was gazing not only on what lay behind us but also on what our future foreshadowed.

I feared I was trapped in the jaws of fear, and I could see no way to shake loose. Faced day in and day out with Martha's decline, I just . . . couldn't . . . shake . . . her symptoms from my mind. *This is hopeless,* I thought. *I can't do this.* I called Jim Glennon for help. "This is hard work, Jim. In fact, it's the hardest thing I've ever tried to do."

"I didn't say it was easy, Carlen. I said it works." I laughed out loud. I was quickly discovering that Jim was one of those classic curmudgeons: crusty on the outside, warm and soft on the inside.

"You might want to talk with Don Jaeger," Jim suggested. "He's over in your corner of the kingdom. Winter Park, I believe. Don was diagnosed with ALS. I believe you in the States call that Lou Gehrig's disease. He's now completely healed."

ALS is a degenerative, fatal disease, according to the medical community. *Just as alzheimer's is a degenerative and ultimately fatal disease,* I thought. *Maybe there's hope yet.*

So in the fall of 1999, two years after Martha's diagnosis, I called Don Jaeger, and we later met in Winter Park. Don was mobile and healthy except for a slight limp, and I was skeptical that he'd ever suffered from Lou Gehrig's disease. I thought he'd been misdiagnosed. This is his story as I pieced it together from our conversations. About seven years earlier, Don was diagnosed with ALS by a local neurologist and an EMG specialist; and this was later confirmed by a leading neurologist at the University of Florida's Shands Hospital. (Don makes his medical records available for anyone caring to see them, he told us.)

Don is an entrepreneur, and I know through operating my business magazine that the successful ones are not inclined to wishful thinking or excessive words. Don's a *Dragnet* Sgt. Friday kind of guy: "Just the facts, ma'am."

He says his Episcopal pastor suggested he attend a healing conference nearby with Canon Glennon, where they prayed for his healing. He followed Jim's suggestion to turn away from his symptoms and fears and turn toward the fullness of God's kingdom.

He and his wife prayed to see God in all this, he said. "The toughest part I faced was the fear of the disease's onslaught, and of leaving my family."

While waiting in a doctor's office, a deep certainty came over Don that he no longer had ALS. His skin temperature rose quickly and a peace came over him. "Even Sarah said she saw it." Six months after his initial diagnosis, doctors at the Cleveland Clinic, which specializes in ALS, put Don through an additional battery of tests. A lead physician there told him: "I see more than 150 cases of ALS a year, and you neither have nor show signs of ever having had ALS disease."

Those conversations with Don encouraged me. I understood that the approach to healing as described by Jim Glennon offered no guarantees. But I also understood that with alzheimer's the medical community offered no hope. So I recommitted to Jim's approach. I tried to allow God's kingdom of life and love to reshape who I was, to reconfigure my deepest instincts and feelings.

Why Ask for What You've Got?

I made a measure of progress over the next couple of years—until that fateful day in early June 2002, when Martha fell into that seizure.

That set me back, all the way back. Only two other events had brought me this near to collapse—Martha's diagnosis and my having to take her car keys away. After her seizure I decided to visit Jim in person. *I've got to look him in the eye when we talk,* I thought. *I've got to see for myself what's going on at this healing center.*

I called Jim and told him about Martha's seizure. "When can you see me if I come visit you?"

"Carlen, you don't need to come here. It's too far. I can't tell you any more than I have already."

"I appreciate all you've done so far, Jim. But something is urging me to come see you in person."

"All right, let me check my calendar." The next day he wrote that he could see me the week of July 7–13, 2002.

I left St. Petersburg on the fifth of July to get to Sydney on the seventh. After a layover in Los Angeles, the plane chased the setting sun for fifteen hours. The Pacific Ocean is a big, big tub of water. With little sleep, I stumbled off the plane, picked up my bag, and caught a taxi to the retreat center. Jim left a note saying he would meet me at ten o'clock sharp the next morning. I showered and fell asleep.

I ate breakfast with a handful of guests and staff. The center, I discovered, had been a Catholic convent that the healing ministry purchased several years earlier. After breakfast, the receptionist suggested I wait for Jim in a large drawing room downstairs. I found a comfortable chair and sat down. The room was unlit except for the morning sun, a patchwork of light and shadow dancing across the floor.

The door opened, and Jim entered in a wisp of movement, greeting me with, "Hello, Carlen. I'm Jim Glennon."

I promptly stood and shook his hand. "Jim, it's good to finally meet you in person." I'd seen a picture of him but that didn't come close to conveying the presence that quickly filled this oversized room. We both sat down, Jim in a chair opposite mine.

"Why have you come, Carlen?"

That puzzled me. I thought I'd made that clear on the phone. I fumbled for an answer. "I guess I want to understand this kingdom of God idea, Jim. I need to see it firsthand, I think."

Silence. Jim said nothing. More silence. In a wink, this was no normal, social conversation. I found it difficult to catch Jim's eye. I thought he was looking at me, and then not. *Maybe it's his age,* I thought. He was eighty-two, of my parents' generation. I learned later he had a glass eye. We sat in silence for what must have been fifteen minutes, maybe more. I felt his complete concentration on me, as if taking my measure. I squirmed.

Jim at last broke the spell with a story. "Why ask for what you've got? I puzzled long and hard over that question, Carlen." He first heard it from a couple whose young daughter had a severe case of scoliosis, a sideways curvature of the spine that could affect the function of her lungs. Her prospect for growing into adulthood was dismal at best, the doctors told the couple. She likely would be disabled for life. The couple went to their pastor, asking if the church had a healing ministry that could help. Their minister told them no, there was not. The couple decided to study the New Testament for themselves, highlighting all of Jesus's healings and his references to the kingdom of God. They began to focus their prayers and thoughts on God's gifts and promises rather than on their daughter's problems. When Jim met the couple many years later, their daughter had grown into young adulthood, and her spine was fully straightened.

They told Jim they were guided by three foundational ideas:

- *The perfection is within you.*
- *Why ask for what you've got?*
- *You have what you accept.*

This, they told him, is the essence of Jesus's teachings on the kingdom of God. It was a long while, Jim said, before he grasped what they meant.

I've already heard this story, I thought. *At least half a dozen times. Isn't there a fresh insight he can share?* We nonetheless continued our conversation. Jim sketched out his week's plans for me, for which he would serve as both a spiritual guide and tour director. "You've had a long flight, Carlen. Why don't you relax today? And then we'll go at it tomorrow." He left as quietly as he came.

I went to my room. Jim's comments, though thoughtful, were a repeat of what I'd heard on his tapes, read in his books, and discussed with him by phone. I asked myself the same question Jim asked me earlier: *Why have you come, Carlen?* As I puzzled on that, I realized that this story of the couple and their daughter was clearer to me with this hearing. I sensed that Jim's message of God's kingdom and forgiveness was boring deeper into my thinking.

The next day Jim picked me up and showed me some of the typical tourist spots, such as Sydney's iconic opera house and its famous surfing beaches. Sydney is a city of striking beauty, rivaling that of San Francisco in many ways. Our conversations that day were a casual let's-get-to-know-each-other kind. Throughout the week, he arranged for us to meet with friends over meals, friends who had been healed in their own right. After talking with a couple of them, I noticed a pattern. Jim introduced us and then sat back, his ego tucked away, saying very little while I listened to his friends' comments.

On Wednesday evening, I visited a weekly healing service at St. Andrew's Cathedral in the heart of Sydney. Jim didn't attend because, I surmised, he didn't want his presence to disrupt the leader's agenda. Jim had started and led that ministry for nearly three decades before retiring. The service format included contemporary devotional songs, prayers, readings from the Bible, a short message, and then breaking up into small groups to listen to those in need of healing and to pray with them. I sat on the perimeter of a couple of these groups to watch and listen.

The next day at noon, I went with Jim to a healing service he was leading in Australia's oldest Catholic church, St. Mary's Cathedral. It was quieter with fewer people in attendance than the previous night. Standing before three dozen folks in the gray, cavernous nave of this nineteenth-century Gothic structure, Jim again discussed God's kingdom and its many provisions.

"If you're fighting with your problems, you're already on the losing side," he emphasized. I was reminded of all my wrestling with Martha's symptoms and the fear they engendered.

On my last full day in Sydney, I was stirred awake early in the morning. I recorded what transpired in my journal:

JULY 13, 2002

I awoke at three o'clock this morning, praying: "My dear Father, this is why I came to Sydney. You've permitted me finally to know that your kingdom is perfect and complete in every way—no sin, no suffering, no sickness, not even any alzheimer's. Your kingdom is replete with love, trust, hope, and wholeness. As we go forward, I ask you to lead us away from the temptation to focus on the symptoms that have severely tested us. Deliver us from the evil that says we are without hope.

I stopped breathing. That's interesting . . . without realizing it I had adapted the final statements of the Lord's Prayer to our plight: "Lead us not into temptation . . . deliver us from evil." I wondered, What would happen if I start at the beginning of this prayer?

"Our Father who art in heaven, hallowed be thy name."

"Yes, Father," a voice responded deep within. "Your name indeed is holy, and you are far removed from our family's problems—far from those forces that seek to devour our family." I cried at the thought of this.

Something jarred me, and in my mind's eye I saw our Father step down from his throne in heaven and unfurl a tent over me. I saw this as clearly as I've ever seen the morning sun. It covered Martha, our children, and me. But this wasn't a tent. Our Father was unfurling his Name over us. I cried aloud, gulping for air. "Thank you, Father," I whispered. "Thank you."

My hand shakes as I write this. My tears stain my

> *pillow. My heart trembles with the thought of You descending over our family. We don't deserve this. We don't deserve such attention. Why have You done this? Why have You unfurled your Most Holy Name over our family?*

Tossing in bed, with the question *why?* echoing in my mind, this answer arose: *My master Christ Jesus pleaded our case. And the God of all creation, the God above all, the living God, has heard. And he has responded.*

I fell asleep, exhausted and spent.

The next morning, I wanted to share this dreamlike encounter with Jim. But I didn't see him all day. He later dropped by as I was eating dinner. Soon, Jim and I had a few private minutes together, and I told him about this early morning encounter. "God has richly blessed you," is all that he said in his quiet, authoritative voice. Then he got up to leave, to catch a bus downtown for a dinner engagement. I walked the couple of blocks with him to King Street. The bus arrived, we shook hands, and Canon Jim Glennon stepped on board and waved good-bye through the window. The next morning I flew home.

Déjà Vu

I enjoyed an afterglow for weeks following my visit. As Jim and I continued to correspond, seemingly minor improvements began to occur with Martha, such as in her ability to go for walks and to get dressed. Before Sydney, these activities were arduous. She resisted any kind of change, large or small, which I learned was typical of a person with alzheimer's. Walking with her around the block for exercise had been like tugging a bag of sand. But after I returned from Sydney, Martha started to relax during these short walks. We walked side by side holding hands rather than with me pulling and urging her onward. Likewise, changing into her nightgown no longer was a wrestling match but an act of ease—what had taken twenty minutes now required one.

It's easy to make a case that my attitude had changed rather than anything within Martha. Frankly, I didn't care who or what changed so long as Martha showed improvement. Meanwhile, she began to display an empathy that I had thought was lost. This is a short note in my journal:

My heart melted this morning before going to work. Martha crawled into bed with Kathryn and hugged her as Kathryn snuggled under her arm. The last few days Martha's disposition has been sweeter than I can remember. And there have been whispers of cognizance that I haven't heard in a long while.

On another occasion, I walked into the house after work, ready to relieve our caregiver. "Hey, Martha and Tricia, what's happening?" Martha was standing behind Tricia as she sat on our couch watching *Oprah*. Martha looked at me, bent forward slightly, and put a finger to her lips for me to be quiet. *What's this?*

I wondered. *Probably something random.* As I came closer I saw Tricia crying. *Oh my, Martha is protecting Tricia.*

Several days later I was moved to tell her, "I love you, Martha." She looked right into my eyes and clearly, with no hesitation or bumbled words, said, "I love you too." I cried.

"We don't say how sick we are by sight; we say how well we are by faith." If I heard that expression once from Jim, I heard it a hundred times. *Stop giving in to the symptoms displayed by Martha,* is how I understood the expression. *And start embracing the presence of God's kingdom within Martha—life, love, intelligence—whether I see any physical signs yet or not.* The changes I saw in Martha were small indeed. Nevertheless, they felt like major advances.

I tried to share this vision of God's kingdom with a handful of people in St. Petersburg, Christian-type folks, and I was met with a variety of responses—from muted encouragement to polite patronizing to outright criticism. I soon discovered that I wasn't ready to field such criticism as old fears reared up—fear of failure, fear of embarrassment, fear of being misunderstood. I felt like the greatest of fools because I was actually seeking Martha's full recovery. "Yesterday was the worst day I've had since Martha's seizure," I wrote in my journal about six weeks after visiting Sydney. "A fear of her relapse grips me. A black hole of anxiety seeks to draw me in."

Regardless, I continued to contact Jim. He picked up quickly on my inability to thank God in an authentic way. "It's not just important to be grateful to God," Jim said. "It's absolutely necessary if you want to see any progress in healing."

Then he added, "It's not uncommon for a time of blessing to be followed by a time of problems." Jim's words usually steadied me, but not now. Despite all I'd seen, despite all I'd received, my fear was running rampant. Nonetheless, I kept at trying to know God's love regardless of my feelings. It was in vain. "I don't think I'm ever going to get this," I wrote Jim. He was sympathetic and told me of his own inadequacies at crucial moments. "We're only human, Carlen." And then he added, "We may like to think healing depends on us, but it doesn't. It depends on God, so we must depend on him."

A year after my trip to Sydney, Martha suffered a second seizure, as severe as the first. With this one, though, I didn't call 911. Instead, I grabbed Martha and sat down on the floor, holding her in my arms. These things seem as if they last an hour, but it's only for a few minutes. There on the floor, I began to thank God that his healing light was flowing through Martha's mind and body—and mine—calming us both, bringing peace where there were convulsions. I continued to picture this in my mind. I didn't try to restrain the convulsions. I relaxed the best I could, cradling her in my lap, keeping her head to the side to prevent her from swallowing too much saliva.

When the seizure ceased, Martha fell into a deep sleep, again almost coma-like. After lifting her onto the bed, I sat beside her, holding her hand. I continued to see God's light—to *receive* God's light—as it flowed through both her and me. Martha slept much of that day. By the next morning, she was up and about as though nothing had happened—what a marked contrast to the hospital scene following her first seizure. As for me, I was neither exhausted nor wrenched by the chaotic fear I had felt during that first seizure. With the onset of this seizure, and for some time afterward, I felt as though Martha and I were immersed in a bath of love and trust. I continued to thank God while this thought streamed through my mind: *Everything's all right, Carlen; everything's all right.*

PART THREE

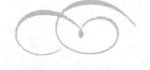

THE WAY OF INTIMACY

EIGHT

A CREEK RUNS THROUGH IT

But we know, in some moments of our lives, what life is.
We know that it is great and holy, deep and
abundant, ecstatic and sober, limited and
distorted by time, fulfilled by eternity.

—Paul Tillich, *The Eternal Now*

As a boy, I loved to roam over my grandfather's farm, which in those days stood a few miles out in the country, south of my small hometown of Cookeville, Tennessee. Today, it's crisscrossed with city streets. Pigeon Roost farm had been in the family from 1925 until 2014, when it was sold. It had open pastures, lots of woods, fields of corn and hay and tobacco, a log smokehouse, several barns and sheds, a few good hills to climb, an oversized garden, some caves and sinkholes, milk cows, mules, chickens, pigs, and a kennel of foxhounds. We lived in town, but my family still got our milk, eggs, butter, and bacon from this farm that Dad grew up on. We knew winter had passed when our sips of fresh milk reeked of wild onions.

A creek tumbled down through the belly of the farm a hundred yards behind my grandparents' house. I walked to that creek by opening a wide gate into the barnyard where the cows and mules and pigs hung out—and where the cow pies and occasional snake made me keep a sharp eye on where I stepped. A couple of different paths sloped down from the barnyard to the creek. Its headwater tumbled from a narrow-mouthed cave. From there it swirled over rocks and roots, with some water flowing through a pump and up to a tank standing above the white, antebellum-style house. I can still hear that pump: *thump-thump, thump-thump, thump-thump*. Pigeon Roost Creek was the heart of Grandpa's farm.

The creek provided water to the barn and the house. When I took a bath there, I knew the creek was flooding if muddy water burst out of the faucet. My older brother was six when my parents couldn't find him in our grandparents' house nor outside in the yard. They finally found him sitting beside the ice-cold creek, with half of his clothes off, according to Mom, who laughed as she told me this story. "What are you doing, Bobby?" she asked. "I'm waiting for the water to turn hot," he said, "so I can take a bath."

The creek also was my refuge. I once took a new path to it, climbing over a wire fence and stepping blindly into a bush swarming with yellow jackets. Their stings felt like snake bites until I ran and plopped into the creek, a long hop, skip, and jump away. On hot days I loved taking my shoes off and wading knee-deep through the running water. And when summer turned to fall, I launched flotillas of leaves at the top of the creek until time stood still, watching them float past the pump and drop out of sight over a small waterfall.

Our family's creek mirrors the stream that I sense arises within me. Like the creek, this stream tumbles out from somewhere deep within. I'm not always aware of its movement, but I do know when this stream soaks into the dry, crusty ground of my heart. I feel it too as it falls into stagnant pools of thought, stirring them afresh. This stream—this Christ-stream—upends heavy, emotion-laden rocks to which I'm otherwise blind. Christ knew of my need, hidden from me, to forgive Martha's parents long before my week's stay in Thomas Merton's cabin. He also knew of my desperate thirst for God's love—and Dad's—well ahead of my encounter with Elvis, Dad, and Jesus.

As a boy, I knew Pigeon Roost Creek must have flowed somewhere, but I never gave it any thought. Similarly, I'm unsure where this Christ-stream goes when it spills out from me. However, I do sense that after flowing through my feelings, thoughts, memories, and dreams—transforming the forgotten and remembered, the fractured and whole—this stream then pours out into an ever-greater presence.

An Invitation

In 2002, four-odd years after Martha's diagnosis, I picked up my office phone to hear a brusque voice on the other end of the line: "Carlen, we need to talk." *This has got to be Lacy.* Nobody else I knew had this South Carolina drawl. Rev. Lacy Harwell was the retired Presbyterian minister and friend who was a continual, significant guide during our crisis.

"Hey, Lacy. I can talk now."

"No, no. We've got to talk in person."

I agreed to meet and said, "You want to give me a heads-up on what this is about?"

"Carlen, I said we need to talk in person."

The conversation left me scratching my head. From his tone I thought someone was in trouble, and I wondered if that someone was me.

Lacy and I met for lunch at Demens Landing, a quiet city park looking out over the expanse of Tampa Bay. On one side, sailboats and yachts of all sizes and shapes filled a marina basin. On the other, small private planes flew in and out of a downtown airport. Behind us was St. Petersburg's skyline. A light breeze blew off the bay as a few clouds hung above us on this pleasant winter day.

We sat opposite each other on a concrete picnic table. He began to pray in the humblest whisper I'd heard, "Father, this is Lacy." I almost burst out laughing. His tone and posture of abject humility stood in such marked contrast to his outsized public image. Lacy then proceeded to converse with God with an intimacy I hadn't heard since Martha's putting the kids to bed.

Lacy took a big bite from his sandwich, and while chewing said, "Here's why I called you, Carlen." Skipping small talk suited me fine because the urgency of the matter puzzled me. "Every so often I need to get away for a few hours and wrestle things out with myself and God," Lacy said. "That's what I did a few days ago. I went out to the Sunshine Skyway bridge, as I usually do in moments like this. It was a wet, cold, and messy day. The dark clouds swirling above began to intensify and to brighten. As I watched this phenomenon I heard a voice come from within. There was no audible sound, nor did I see anything physical. But the voice was clear. It spoke in that vocabulary unique to the heart." I recounted what I heard Lacy say in my journal:

> *"Lacy, you have struggled your whole life with questions about suffering. A number of your friends have suffered in untold ways, as have many others under your pastoral care. Their suffering often seemed to have reached no satisfactory resolution. Satisfactory at least to you and your friends."*
>
> *"I am going to tell you, Lacy, all you need to know about suffering, all you can bear to know for now. I too suffer as my children do. Even more. You and your fellow man may think I sit high above all that you experience. I do not. I sent my Son to let you know that I understand what you're going through. It's very important that you pay attention, Lacy, and get this right. All your suffering, all your friends' suffering, will ultimately dissolve into my utter, complete joy. Until then you must not become captive to your suffering or theirs. You must permit me to capture you with my grace and my comfort."*

Lacy paused for a long spell. All I heard were the waves splashing against the nearby seawall and a few gulls conversing overhead. Tears wet the eyes of this larger-than-life man as he continued: *"'Now, Lacy,' this voice said, 'I want you to reflect on all I have told you. And I want you to go tell Carlen all that you've heard.'"*

I stopped breathing. I said nothing. I could say nothing. I cried deep within, a silent cry as real and palpable as the loudest of wails.

Lacy stood up, shook my hand, and walked to his car, neither of us speaking another word.

I sat awhile, my thoughts frozen in awe. But my feelings were pulled by an undertow of gratitude. *Thank you, Master, for letting me know again that you understand our dilemma. Thank you for singling out Martha, our children, and me for this blessing.* I returned to my office, dispensed with any unfinished business, then walked around downtown before going home. That night after Martha fell asleep, I tried to write in my journal what I had heard Lacy share that day. I couldn't put two sentences together that made sense. So I just jotted down notes. It took me a couple of weeks to digest this encounter before I could put it into a cohesive written account.

I emailed Lacy a copy of my journal entry, thanking him and asking him for feedback. The next day my phone rang. "This is Lacy." He was calling from South Carolina. "Carlen, you missed the most important point of what I said." *I see Lacy got my note,* I said to myself, grinning at his abruptness.

To make sure I didn't miss the mark again, Lacy explained more fully what he had told me a couple weeks earlier: "Jesus had his core disciples, and among those was an inner circle of Peter, James, John, and Andrew. Three women also were counted among the inner circle—Mary, Martha, and Mary Magdalene." Lacy stopped, stressing that he wanted me to understand this. Then he continued, "Jesus drew from this inner circle when he was facing something important, like in the Garden of Gethsemane."

Lacy paused. "Carlen, the voice I heard. . . ." He paused again. "The voice I heard extended a clear invitation for you to join him at Gethsemane."

I was struck dumb. Why I had missed this invitation earlier is beyond me. Regardless, its poignant simplicity now engulfed me.

"Such an invitation cannot be squandered, Carlen. Suffering is an occasion and an invitation to enter into an intimate relationship with the Lord himself. I never understood this before now." Lacy stopped, making sure I heard him. He added that God doesn't cause suffering. And we don't want to go looking for it. But when suffering is upon us, it needs to be reshaped into something meaningful. "By his suffering with Martha and you," he said, "Jesus is inviting you to enter into an intimate relationship with him. To not take advantage of such an invitation would be a great tragedy." I hung up the phone, my body shaking in disbelief.

Months later, I asked Lacy for permission to share this story with others. "Yes, you can, *but . . .*" he said. "But only if you let them know I'm not some religious nut who sees visions and hears voices and runs around spouting half-baked prophecies." *Vintage Lacy*, I chuckled to myself.

A Fitful Response

This invitation from Christ Jesus rumbled through my heart and mind. I didn't know what to do with it. Oddly, I thought of Lewis and Clark. Like them, I was striking out into a vast unknown wilderness, which stirred within me a mixture of anticipation and dread. Anticipation, because of the nature and source of this invitation. Dread, for the same reason. I finally decided to read the Gospel accounts and reflect on Jesus's last days, starting with the Garden of Gethsemane.

A couple of weeks later, I returned to St. Leo for my monthly weekend retreat. I spent most of the weekend in my room or behind the guesthouse in what I'd come to call my hot seat. I spoke with no one. I found a book in the little library, *Life of Christ*, by Archbishop Fulton J. Sheen. I read it and the Gospel accounts slowly and aloud, seeking to let the meaning of the words sink into my heart. This process of reading Scripture that monks call *lectio divina* is not unlike fishing. You cast your line into a quiet spot that holds promise, sit still, and wait. You jiggle your line a bit, sit still, and wait. Sometimes you catch your limit, sometimes not. The following journal excerpt describes what unfolded in my mind's eye:

FEBRUARY 22–24, 2002

My mind and heart are darkened. When I'm able to picture Jesus in this garden, it's like an old silent film where the characters move awkwardly and the scenes are disjointed. The image of me as a young boy pops up. This little kid taps Jesus on the back, as only an innocent, naïve child has the audacity to do. Jesus looks at me with a faint smile and mouths silently, "Shhh, Carlen, watch and listen."

Jesus stands up to meet his accusers in the garden. He holds my hand. I peek behind him and see him holding

> *Martha's little hand too. Martha sees me. We grin at each*
> *other, two kids without a clue as to what's going on. "You*
> *can't understand everything you wish to understand," Jesus*
> *whispers to us both. "But you can trust me in all situations,*
> *no matter how dark they may seem." I walk with Jesus to*
> *the infamous high priest's courtyard. I hear Peter, Jesus's*
> *good friend, deny three times that he knows him. I feel*
> *nothing toward Peter, good or ill, as Jesus's words echo in*
> *my heart: "Trust me . . . trust me . . . trust me."*

Later that night I awoke dripping beads of fear and sweat. I dreamed that I too had denied Jesus. In this dream, peers made clear that they'd lost all respect for me because of my affiliation with Christ and his followers. I thought they were characterizing me as reactionary and dense, lacking in intelligence and sophistication. I had long admired these friends, so I found myself at a crossroad— do I affirm my love for Christ Jesus or do I continue going along to get along? Unwilling to decide, I felt Peter's dilemma in my bones as they melted into wax.

But this wasn't the first time I'd denied Jesus. I recalled another period back in my late twenties, when my mother died. Until her death, Mom kept our family together. Hers was the grace that got our family through its troubles. No other pain hurt like the loss of Mom until Martha's diagnosis. With Mom's death, I thought Jesus had let my family down, or at least he hadn't stepped up, and I didn't get past that resentment for several years. Reflecting on both these denials, which arose from my Mom's death and my peers' supposed disdain, I lay awake in that dark room in St. Leo and worried, *Am I so weak that I too would deny him yet a third time, by not entrusting Martha to him?*

⬤────◆────⬤

Another month passed before I returned to St. Leo, which happened to be the Friday in March before the Christian church's celebration of Palm Sunday. While at home, I tried to reflect on Jesus's invitation to join him in Gethsemane, but my efforts were sketchy as I worked at the magazine and cared for Martha. I hoped that this weekend retreat would give me a clearer idea of what I needed to do. But as soon as I set foot on the monastery grounds, a great weariness overcame me. The fifth anniversary of Martha's diagnosis was approaching, and this realization weighed unusually heavy. Then too, the memory of my sister's death a year earlier lodged in my mind. I vividly saw Alice asleep, knocked out with painkillers, with me sitting at her bedside, touching her arm, and feeling her last breath expire in that Nashville hospital room. These dark images surrounding my wife and my sister made this Palm Sunday weekend especially poignant as I reflected on the upcoming week's events. Two thousand years earlier, Jesus was fingered as a traitor and left to die hanging between two thieves—hanging, as it were, in limbo. *I know that feeling all too well*, I said to myself. Thinking on Martha's condition, Alice's death, and Jesus's execution forged within me a triangle of death and tragedy—a personal "Bermuda Triangle" in which I saw all my efforts at thought, prayer, and solace disappear into the darkness of pain.

I kept to myself at St. Leo. I neither ate nor talked with anyone. I attended none of the brothers' services. I stayed either in my room or in my hot seat behind the guesthouse, and sometimes I walked the grounds. My mind overflowed with questions as this thought kept pulsating: *It's time for God to give me some answers.* I sought an opening into Christ's heart and his invitation. But every effort was stymied. I tried to pray and read and meditate in my room, but the walls closed in on me. *Maybe it would help to sit outside.* It didn't. *Maybe walking will loosen my thoughts.* That didn't help. *Okay, Carlen, try to nap.* My eyes wouldn't shut, and my ears heard every creak in that guesthouse. I tried yet again to read the accounts of Jesus's crucifixion. I tried to draw near to Christ on the cross. I tried to sit beside his body in that tomb. I tried to see myself within the glow of his resurrection. Nothing connected; relief was remiss. The only clarity was an image of my nature—dark and ugly. Exasperated and depressed by the futility of it all, I was reminded of my friend's admonition from years earlier: "Be gentle on yourself, Carlen; be gentle." But even that brought no comfort. This weekend was the hardest three days I'd endured spiritually.

On that Palm Sunday afternoon, during my last hour at the monastery, I heard this within my heart: *My work with you isn't done, Carlen. You must die and go into the tomb with me, and there arise with me. You must do this if you want to follow me.* These words rolled over in my mind. Yet despite this voice's encouragement, I still despaired at ever seeing Martha and our family freed from the bonds of alzheimer's. Finally, I felt a light touch on my heart, then a firmer grip on my body, as though Jesus's arm were holding me steady, keeping me true to his path. Standing to get my bag and to head home, I heard one last whisper: *We need more time, Carlen; we need more time.* Tears streamed from my eyes. My dull, thick heart began to loosen. I hadn't cried since Jesus extended his invitation to join him in Gethsemane two months earlier. *Thank you, Master,* I whispered back.

A Last Visit

A couple of months later in early June, Lacy Harwell visited Martha and me on a Saturday afternoon. The three of us sat downstairs in our living room, Lacy and Martha on the couch and I in a chair opposite them. I shared with Lacy what I'd been experiencing since our conversation four months earlier. When I finished, he asked me one question that shot straight through my heart: "What did you experience on Easter?"

I thought a moment before responding. "Nothing in particular, I guess. I must still be in process." I had gained little strength or insight from the thought of Jesus's resurrection. I tried to seek joy in God's presence, but mostly I was still pained by the disease plaguing Martha, our children, and me.

"You know," said Lacy, "the story of Lazarus kept coming to me during Easter and for weeks after that." Lazarus was the friend whom Jesus raised from the dead, the Gospel account tells us. "You got a Bible around here?"

"I'll run upstairs and get one."

When I handed him the Bible, he said, "Okay to read this to you?"

"Sure." I would listen to anything that might crack open this iron matrix of despair and anxiety.

Lacy flipped the pages to John's Gospel, reading in his slow, deep drawl. He read that Jesus cried, moved deeply by the grief of his friends Mary and Martha over their brother's death. Lacy also read that Jesus ordered the removal of the stone from the tomb's opening. Finally, reading at the top of his voice, as though preaching to a gathering of five hundred, Lacy yelled these words of Jesus: "Lazarus, come out!"

Martha, Lacy, and I slumped back into our seats. We sat still for several minutes. Then he said, "You might want to reflect on this story, Carlen, and on those involved in it." Lacy stood up, hugged Martha, shook my hand, and stepped out the door without saying another word, not even good-bye.

I reflected on this story at home and at work. I tried to step into the roles of the various characters—Jesus, Lazarus, Mary, Martha, the disciples, and the mourners. But I kept returning to Lazarus, as if by default. *That's where the Spirit seems to be taking me—into Lazarus's tomb*, I thought.

I heard the Spirit whisper in my heart, saying that before Christ could call me out, he needed two things: *First, hang with him on the cross until you hear Jesus breathe his last, saying, "It is finished!" Then he wants you to lie in the tomb with him. Don't step away from the cross or the tomb too soon,* the Spirit cautioned my heart. *Wait until you hear the Master call you. Then you will encounter the full embrace of his resurrection and ascension.*

One night a week later, after Martha fell asleep, I sat downstairs in our living room, more relaxed than I'd been in a long while. As I reflected again on this Lazarus story, I heard a loud echo within my heart: *Carlen, come out!* In the silence of this moment I felt as though I were Lazarus—wrapped in the grave clothes of death and disease, my sight decayed, my movement bound, my flesh and bones chilled by fear. Then I felt the unraveling of those clothes as the darkness scattered and the dead air stirred. *Christ is calling me. He's calling me from this sealed tomb of self-absorption,* I thought. His shout rang through my bones. His voice coursed through my heart. I stood. And I wept aloud.

⟫•◦•⟪

One story in the Gospels attributed to Jesus is commonly known as the parable of the sower. As a farmer sows seed for the season's crop, the story goes, the seeds fall onto various types of land—a well-worn path, thorn-infested ground, rocky soil, and a fertile field. I used to think these diverse soils referred to different kinds of people and their receptivity, or lack of receptivity, to God and his Word, which may be true on one level. But as I puzzled over this story, a greater meaning emerged for me. Meditation and spiritual healing had helped burn off enough emotional underbrush that I was beginning to see new patterns. These different soils described by Jesus were the ever-changing states of mind that cropped up within me.

As I thought about this parable, I saw and heard Robert at work plowing on my grandfather's farm. Robert Phillips, who lived with his family on the farm, wasn't driving a big John Deere tractor combine. He was working a single-blade plow pulled by an ol' mule. "Hyah, Kit!" he yelled as he snapped the mule's reins. With that snap, Kit stepped out and the plow lurched forward as it dug into the dirt. They plowed straight ahead for about fifty yards, then Robert jerked the plow around and he and Kit turned up another row roughly parallel to the previous one. Back and forth they plowed until the whole field was ready to be seeded.

That's what Christ Jesus does.

That's what he did when Martha and I met Sr. Elaine and Fr. Matthew, and when I met Canon Jim Glennon. That's what he did when he drew me into the practices of meditation, *lectio divina*, and spiritual healing. That's what he did when he asked me to join him at Gethsemane. Christ set the point of his plow into the raw earth of my consciousness. He plowed across the charred grounds of my spirit. Back and forth, back and forth, back and forth, he was continuing to plow. As he did, he was turning up the rock-strewn fields of my mind. He was turning under the fear-tipped thorns of my heart. He was enriching the soil of my pinched imagination.

He was preparing me for—*what?*

NINE

MARTHA'S SONG

He who bends to himself a joy
Does the winged life destroy;
But he who kisses the joy as it flies
Lives in eternity's sunrise.
—William Blake, "Eternity"

Martha was diagnosed with alzheimer's in 1997; she entered the Menorah Manor nursing home a decade later. After countless hours of sitting silently together in her room there, holding hands, trying to let her know she was not alone, I sensed a song rising from deep within Martha. It was a quiet song, not even a whisper, that I heard within my heart. This song gently filled Martha's room, caressing her as it caressed me. Her agitation ceased; my mind's chatter halted. This sacred song had everything to do with God's commitment to Martha and her well-being—and to our children and their families, as well as to me.

Martha's song echoed back to our visit with Mary and Paul Zahl, about three years after her diagnosis. The Zahls introduced us to Janice and Peter Newton, who led a healing ministry at Paul's Episcopal church in downtown Birmingham. In the process of becoming acquainted, Janice out of the blue mentioned that she had "the gift of tongues and interpretation." Martha and I looked askance at each other, our eyes narrowing. Our limited experience with this kind of "gift" had left us both cold. The expression on Martha's face seemed to form a question: *What are we doing here?*

Janice apparently picked up on our skepticism and moved the conversation along to other subjects, helping to put us both more at ease. Soon, though, Janice turned to Martha and said, "I feel this gift's movement within me. Would it be okay if I share this with you?"

Martha looked at me. I looked back at her. Martha took a deep breath, nodded, and whispered, "Yes."

What followed is all but indescribable, even to this day. We gathered in a circle, seated, heads bowed as in prayer: Janice, Peter, Mary, Martha, and me. Janice spoke in an unintelligible language; her voice had an angelic tone and melody. As she talked, a sense of peace settled over our small circle, a silence that I can only describe as a lyrical holiness. Have you ever been so deep in a forest that you heard not one sound, then suddenly from afar a bird began to sing? That's what it felt like. We opened our eyes, and Janice said she would interpret this revealed message. She asked Peter to write it down:

MAY 13, 2000

Martha, you have been walking through a mist, through a dark cloud. But you have kept walking, and that is very important.

I have walked beside you, Martha, so that you would not lose the way. The path has not been an aimless one. You have never lost the way even though you have felt that you have been stumbling against rocks strewn in your path.

If you have wanted to take your hand away from mine, you have never done that.

If you have been tempted to stop walking, you have always kept going.

The pressure to deny me has been strong, but the strength of your faith has been stronger, and you have never denied me.

What a beloved child you are to me. Where others would have collapsed in the face of despair, you, my beloved Martha, have never denied me.

I love you for your steadfastness. And in your weakness I hold you close to me like an infant. You will keep walking, holding my hand. You will not be lost to me.

So I bless you. I bless you. I bless you with my touch. I bless you with my strength.

Together we walk into the future, and together we will be strong.

Nothing can stand in my way. I am the Lord and I have declared my Name, which is eternal.

Martha and I, hand in hand, wept quietly. I whispered to myself, *This is the gift of a divine voice—not "of tongues."*

I don't know whether such a gift is unique to the Christian faith. I suspect it's not. Many gifts and practices that I once thought were unique to Christianity I've since discovered are in other faiths as well. After all we've been through, I've come to understand that God respects and loves us all, regardless of where we are in our faith.

Of all that's been revealed to Martha and me, of all the good and bad we've endured along this path, of all our suffering and the blessings, this divine voice stands apart. It stands sure and firm in my memory, a song lifted in a clear, pure voice. This blessing is a climactic note in Martha's legacy.

As we sat in her nursing home, silently holding hands, this song's blessing enfolded Martha and me. Arising from this silent bond, I heard these words: *As this blessing was given unto Martha, she now gives it to her children, and to her children's children, and to their children.*

Martha's legacy echoes through this song as it unfolds through David, Rachel, and Kathryn, and through their families. Now in his early forties, David tells me how much he enjoys and needs his swimming workouts, and I think back to when Martha forced him, over fuss and fury, to try out for his high school swim team. And Rachel, a teacher of English as a second language, takes her mother's love for teaching to the college level. Kathryn, both as a child and as an adult, always has displayed an independent streak and an empathy for society's underdogs that so marked Martha's character. I see Martha dancing in our children's eyes and hear her laugh ringing in theirs. Martha's love and care for children streams through our children—the tenderness and attention shown by David and Rachel with their own, and by Kathryn not only with her nephews and nieces but also through her profession of working with foster kids and displaced families.

Martha and I have kept this song, which was revealed through Janice, hidden long enough, too long really. As I read it yet again, its crystalline message and melody flow over me. And I'm reminded of Jesus's words: "Nor do men light a lamp and put it under a bushel, but on a stand, and it gives light to all in the house" (Matt. 5:15).

Although Martha was unable to say this in any perceptible way, I know within our silent bond that this would have been her desire: *This song of divine grace was given to me, so I give it to you. It's my gift to anyone who hears it and who seeks it for his or her own.*

If there's a whisper of meaning in this prayer-song for you, then stop. Read it aloud slowly, softly, again and again. Accept this gift from Martha, replacing her name with yours. Then let your heart sink into it, and sing this prayer-song aloud until you make it your own.

Embrace this blessing with the grace and light and dignity by which it was given to Martha.

Embrace it in Christ's love; embrace it in Martha's love.

For this is his gift and hers to you. And if you do receive it, then do as Martha would do—pass it on to another.

Selah.

REPORTING BACK

The wilderness and the dry land shall be glad. . . .
For waters shall break forth in the wilderness,
and streams in the desert. . . .
And a highway shall be there, and it shall
be called the Holy Way.

—Isaiah 35:1, 6, 8

Out of the Wilderness

Only recently has the meaning of my walk with Martha at Gethsemani come clear to me, carved out like a statue in relief by the intervening years. In so many ways this walk in 1997 foreshadowed what was to come. Our family has stepped over jutting rocks and tangled roots and moved through a wooded darkness speckled with light. We have stumbled onto sunlit clearings and paused at the wonder of it all, lingering with delight before turning back to the path set before us. Yes, ours has been a maddening and frustrating journey, disheartening even. Yet somehow this walk—our walk—has followed a sacred path, pointing our way toward a Presence far greater and more real than any entrapment by a disease.

In his book *Darling: A Spiritual Autobiography*, Mexican-American essayist Richard Rodriguez set out to explore a fuller understanding of his faith's birthplace and its relation to Islam. Catholic from birth, Rodriguez says his autobiography was precipitated by 9/11's tragic events. He knew, as did I, that his Christian faith has a father in common with Islam and Judaism—Abraham. But not until reading *Darling* did it dawn on me that the three faiths also share the same mother—the barren desert. I'm not a student of world religions, but as I turned this over in my mind, I wondered how many of the world's long-standing faiths arose from a wasteland or wilderness of some kind—the desert, a barren mountain range, the dark jungle.

It then struck me that a more authentic and intimate faith often must arise out of some personal wasteland: the premature loss of a parent, spouse, or child; irreversible illness; depression or another emotional disability; financial collapse—you name it. But I may be painting with too broad a brush, so let me scale back to our story. My faith was fabricated from a variety of authoritative voices telling me what I should or should not believe. Then one day Martha and I awoke to find ourselves in the middle of a desert. When you're lost in a vast desert, the choices you face are few, all stark: sit down and die, run helter-skelter to nowhere, or search for water. We went searching.

This impulse to search drove me to places I'd never thought of going—monasteries and spiritual mentors, meditation and spiritual healing. These were foreign, some even heretical, to my religious upbringing. But when modern medicine had no answer but death by slow attrition, I had little choice but to look elsewhere. Had I not, I may well have sunk into despair or cynicism, ultimately letting Martha and the children fend for themselves. And where would they be today? Or I?

As I began trying to sort the credible from the dubious, this thought occurred to me: How much of this universe does modern science truly have a fix on? Ten percent? Five percent? I'm told five percent is overly generous. Regardless, starting with medicine's modest knowledge of alzheimer's and its causes, I set out to explore to the best of my limited abilities the ninety-five percent that science and medicine do not yet know. I explored not merely in a rational, intellectual way, but emotionally and spiritually as well. Science has barely explored our human consciousness, both individual and collective. Just what is its role in shaping and defining the condition of our bodies? Our physical environment? What is its impact on the well-being of our families, communities, and nations? A major reason human consciousness remains unexplored by science is the virtual impossibility of measuring and monitoring it in a meaningful way.

If you've ever looked into the metaphysics of consciousness, you've no doubt come across this question: Which is real—physical matter or spirit? But that's the wrong question, at least for me at this stage in my understanding. The better one to ask is this: Which do I let inform my character, identity, and instincts—my fickle mind and inconstant physical senses, or the Spirit's deep, abiding presence?

It seems to me that Jesus answers this when he says, "Seek first [God's] kingdom and his righteousness" (Matt. 6:33). This is the principle by which Canon Jim Glennon instructed me to focus not on losses or gains with Martha's symptoms, but on the character of God.

"Once you glimpse God's kingdom," Jim said, "be grateful for what you've received, whether little or large. You need to reach the point where your gratitude is full-hearted and full-throated." I found that hard to do, even impossible at times. Yes, I could fake it, but feeling thankful deep within was difficult as I watched Martha slip further away month by month. Yet I found lasting value in even attempting to thank God in an honest way.

The Kingdom Is Come. Really?

A friend asked me not long ago what I've been doing since 2002. I was surprised by her question, because I hadn't recognized that year marked a turning point when the string of dramatic encounters I've described began to diminish. I now realize that in the ensuing years I've tried to understand, appreciate, and rely on God's character in a richer, fuller, more instinctive manner, fleshing out Canon Glennon's words: *The perfection is within you. Why ask for what you've got? You have what you accept.*

His emphasis on the "kingdom of God" confused me initially. My mind conjured up images of autocratic regimes, armies, geographic territories, and massive wealth. I couldn't connect these images with the healing of body, mind, and soul. But gradually

I came to understand what Christ Jesus meant. This kingdom is charged with God's nature—love, courage, spirit, humility, clarity of mind, strength, persistence, wholeness, boldness, mercy, transparency, and confidence. It lies within each of us, but as a dormant seed until we recognize it and let Christ call out its hidden strength, qualities, and beauty.

As my understanding of God's kingdom deepened, my grasp of Jesus's statement sharpened: "No one can serve two masters" (Matt. 6:24). *I cannot keep waffling. Either I focus on Martha's symptoms, or I focus on God's kingdom and righteousness. I can't do both.* I finally decided to focus on this spiritual kingdom even though it would have been so much easier to stay focused on the symptoms and let them victimize me.

This refocusing caused me to see something else for the first time: Jesus's commandment to "seek first the kingdom" isn't just some sermon topic. Rather, it's a hard-won insight by which Christ Jesus taught, acted, and healed. It's the axis around which his life revolved. It's the prism through which he viewed the world, distinguishing reality from illusion. It's the force by which he arose from the grave.

Practically speaking, what does God's kingdom mean when you're trapped in a crisis like ours? Early on, Martha's symptoms made me want to crawl under my sheets and never come out. Those sheets were soaked in fear—fear of losing Martha, fear of failing our children, fear of losing myself. I let these fears enshroud me with darkness. Eventually I saw that long before Martha's illness I had suppressed all kinds of negative feelings—resentment, fear of disease and death, arrogance, anger, depression, and self-righteousness. Cemented over time, such fears assume a reality of their own, often playing out in aching joints, heart palpitations, constipation, headaches, upset stomach, or almost any form of illness.

If I try to fight such mind-sets, I lose; if I give in to them, I also lose. The more I wrestled, the more I saw that these deep-seated feelings were my worst enemy. As I recognized this, Jesus's command streamed through my mind: "Love your enemies." *Huh? How can I love that which I hate?* In the midst of this turmoil, it dawned on me: *If I want to be freed, I must permit God's love, not mine, to overcome these dark feelings.*

Why Not?

God continues to show our children and me that a wasting disease does not have to define who we are. *You are not a tragedy called alzheimer's. You are perfect and whole within our Father's heart and mind.*

And yet, I've asked myself many times, *if that's true, why hasn't Martha returned to a normal, natural state of mind and body?* And ultimately my answer is: *I don't know.* Through the years, a sweetness emerged within Martha and in our relationship. But I haven't seen all that I hoped for and expected when I set out on this path. I've talked with enough people who were physically healed by spiritual means to know it happens. I've talked with others who were diligent and faithful and not healed. When I discussed this with Jim Glennon, he acknowledged that, while not all were healed through his ministry, not all are healed through traditional medicine either. "But, Carlen, every single person who embarked on a path of spiritual healing has expressed gratitude for the richness of meaning and understanding they have gained."

And so do I.

Friends have shared with me a question they've heard from others, but one I've never been asked directly: why, or how, have I continued to visit Martha day in and day out, five to six days a week, even though she can't walk, can't talk, can't feed herself, and rarely recognizes me? My response: "Because Martha is still a person. And she's still my girlfriend and our children's mother."

I'm convinced that Martha was attuned to the Spirit's movement, despite symptoms that restricted any visible expression of faith. When I would show up in her room at Menorah Manor, Martha often was agitated, tossing and turning in her chair or bed. I would touch her and she might jerk away. "Hi Martha," I'd say. "This is me, Carlen." Sometimes my voice would give pause to her agitation, sometimes not. I would usually say a few more words. "I saw David's children this weekend. You'd love Libby and Nelson and Bennett. And Rachel's little girl, Olivia, was asking all about her Mimi the other day. That's you, Martha; you're Mimi." Then I'd sit down beside her and slowly work my hand into hers, which often was clenched into a fist. Soon, our hands would relax within each other's. I would sit quietly. I'd envision our Christ spreading his cloak of humility over us both. Often, a stillness from somewhere beyond Martha and me would descend on us. Martha's body would calm; my heart and mind would relax.

I sense that this was Christ's presence, but I can't prove it. However, in no other setting have I more consistently felt this peaceful presence than when I was sitting there with Martha, being still, holding her hand.

I remember one Sunday at church, a couple of years before

Martha moved into the nursing home. There was little about the service with which Martha seemed to connect. But when we stood to sing "Amazing Grace," tears streamed down Martha's cheeks. I looked into her eyes, which often were clouded with confusion. She looked back at me but didn't see me. She was looking far beyond me, her blue eyes clear and bright. I needed no other sign to know that she was somewhere else, embraced in a dance sweet and intimate.

An Intimate Way

My struggle to focus on the attributes of God's kingdom echoes my struggle to follow Jesus's charge in Mark's Gospel: "And you shall love the Lord your God with all your heart, and with all your soul, and with all your mind, and with all your strength" (Mk. 12:30).

I wrestled with that directive long before Martha's illness. I tried to obey it but felt no emotional oomph. Through my encounters with Christ, however, it finally dawned on me that trying to love an all-powerful, all-knowing, all-seeing, infinite, invisible, perfect being we call God is futile. Seeking to understand why and how God loves me has proved much more fertile. I realized—and oh, this came so slowly—that Jesus's command mirrors God's commitment to me. The more I recognize this fact, the easier I'm able to respond in similar fashion.

I can love God only to the degree that I know God loves me.

I can humble myself before God only to the point that I see God's humility expressed toward me.

I can trust God only to the extent that I realize I've been entrusted with God's Name and image.

And I can enjoy God only to the depth that I feel God's joy for me.

In other words, I'm able to heed Jesus's command with all that I am only when I know and feel deep within that God loves me with all his heart, soul, mind, and strength. And only then do I understand that this command is not a command at all. It's a promise: "You *shall* love the Lord your God." This love is not sentimental. It is the perfect, complete love that makes us whole, knitting our bodies, minds, and spirits into the One.

I encountered such divine intimacy in March 2014 in, of all places, a hotel room in Macon, Georgia. I was on a road trip with our daughter Rachel and her two-year-old daughter, Olivia Grace. I was reflecting on the opening words of an ancient psalm that offered me a measure of comfort, though I had never grasped its meaning: "He that dwelleth in the secret place of the most High shall abide under the shadow of the Almighty" (Ps. 91:1 KJV).

Right before dawn, Olivia's tiny voice awakened me: "Mommie . . . Mommie . . . Mommie." I opened my eyes to see a crescent moon and stars on the darkened ceiling. It was a bedtime toy to help comfort Olivia. I saw Rachel bending over Olivia in her bed, but saw none of Rachel's features, not even her flaming red hair. All I could see was the silhouette of a mother silently hovering over her child, touching her head, checking her diaper, pulling up the sheets, whispering words only her child can hear.

Seeing this intimate moment, I thought: *So this is what it means to "abide under the shadow of the Almighty."* During the darkest of hours this Shadow hovered over Martha, mothering

her, caressing her, protecting her, singing to her, whispering in her
ear. As with Martha, this Shadow hovers over me too, and over
our children, and over their children.

———————————

As I reflect on our family's remarkable odyssey, I see that my
encounters with Christ Jesus are expressions of God's nature, or
kingdom. I couldn't have planned or anticipated these encounters.
My week in Thomas Merton's cabin, for instance, made clear that,
if I wanted to be made whole, I needed to forgive Martha's parents.
My reflection on my memory of rocking out like Elvis in front of
Dad lifted a lifelong barrier to trust and intimacy. In Sydney, my
walled emotions broke loose when I saw our Father unfurl his
Name over Martha, over our children, and over me. And finally,
when Christ invited me into the darkness of that garden called
Gethsemane, I was deeply, fearfully humbled.

A good friend tells me that people reading about my vivid
encounters with God may wonder what I was smoking. We had
a good laugh—I think he was laughing with me. They were not
hypnotic trances. They were not like an athlete envisioning his
swing of the bat or throw of the football. Those are self-directed.
My experiences were not. My role was to be still and open to
God's presence as best I could. This sometimes took days, if not
weeks or months, as I went about my regular business. But at
some point, all control was lifted from me and I felt my heart
and mind become one, clear of distraction and interference. An
atmosphere of humility and vulnerability enfolded me, and the
encounters I've described arose unexpectedly, flowing through my

mind, memory, and heart.

I've drawn one undergirding lesson from these moments: the goal is not a dramatic, emotional encounter, so I don't seek it. Well, I do sometimes, but when I do I realize its futility yet again. Instead, I ask God to release his humility, spirit, mind, and love deep within me. They are rooted in each of us. In other words, I thank him for the promise that "the kingdom of heaven is at hand" (Matt. 3:2). Then I wait for a response. Whatever arises, whether dramatic or ordinary, will be sufficient. My object, I now understand, is to permit God's intimate touch to disrupt and enrich all that I believe, think, feel, and do, all that I am—body and soul, heart and mind.

It took a long while before I understood this fundamental fact: God has given each of us the spiritual resources and framework to face a crisis that seeks to crush us. We are created with the capacity to discover these resources. And as we do, we must be willing to embrace them. I continue to learn almost daily from Jesus's teachings and actions that I am not—as you are not—separate from God. I am—as you are—an expression of God's love, an expression of God's life, and an expression of God's mind and spirit. This understanding is as ancient as the stars, yet its impact on me continues to be revolutionary. When I encountered Christ Jesus through these years of struggle, the moments often faded into a lingering question: *Now, Carlen, do you know our Father loves you? Loves Martha? David, Rachel, Kathryn?* Little by little, I got it. Encounter by encounter, this realization of God's thirst for my intimacy took hold in the core of my consciousness. It continues to.

Before feeling such intimacy, I often ricocheted between the rails of willfulness and willingness, as Sr. Elaine had called me out on. Eventually I learned that willfulness is driven by fear, while willingness is grounded in faith. I used to think faith meant holding tight to a system of beliefs, asserting their values over all else. Faith instead is a movement from darkness to light, from fractured to whole. Faith is a profound intimacy, allowing me to be wrapped in Christ's cloak of humility as he whispers: *Rest for awhile, Carlen. Be gentle on yourself. We have enough time to accomplish the work ahead.*

The Christ called Jesus whom I now know does not carry a list of moralistic and theological bullet points, or institutional creeds and confessions. Nor does he offer some formulaic salvation. Rather, he reveals to me a path previously hidden, by which he invites me to walk with him into the deep we call God. On this path, he guides me homeward to our Father's face of humility and joy. Christ Jesus holds my hand, cajoles me, lets me cook in my juices, walks before me, walks behind me, drags me, stations guides along my way, picks me up, appears in my imagination, whispers in my ear, laughs with me, loves me, trusts me, heals me.

A MOM AND HER CHILDREN

Truly, I say to you, unless you turn and become like
children, you will never enter the kingdom of heaven.

—Jesus, Matthew 18:3

To be a child of Martha's you have to like
Montreat, tennis, and grits.

—Kathryn, Rachel, and David

"**M**ommie used to say she didn't want us to be wallflowers
when we grew up." Kathryn recalls being picked up from
grade school, the radio blaring with the Beatles or some other
oldie. Martha would place her hand on Kathryn's while keeping
time to the music. "That definitely embarrassed me as I got older."
Especially with her friends in the back seat. "She wanted to make

sure I 'had rhythm.' I had to learn how to sing, but particularly how to dance."

Years after Kathryn's rhythm lessons, our children were stepping into young adulthood when Martha was diagnosed with alzheimer's. David was a twenty-two-year-old senior at Davidson College in North Carolina; Rachel, twenty, was a sophomore at the University of North Carolina; and Kathryn was sixteen, still at home and a junior at St. Petersburg High. They, like me, had given no thought to alzheimer's before it afflicted their mother. *Old people worry about alzheimer's, not someone Martha's age,* I recall thinking. My heart sank as I soon realized that the strong, comforting mother they grew up loving probably would not be there much longer. And it dawned on me that as a parent I'd be taking on more than I'd planned for.

Our story would be incomplete without our children's voices, feelings, and insights. The following is drawn from conversations with each of them. The contrasts are sharp and vivid between our children's memories prior to the diagnosis (*shown in italics*) and their thoughts about their mother over her last seventeen years.

Singing 'n' Dancing

Our children say they can still hear their mother's voice at bedtime. Martha rubbed their backs while singing all kinds of songs to them, from rock to country, pop to religious.

"I cry every time I hear the Lord's Prayer sung," says Kathryn. She remembers her mother hitting its high notes perfectly—"for thine is the kingdom, and the power, and the glory forever."

Rachel recalls walking up to our house hearing her mother's voice belting out a tune from the kitchen. "Your mom's always singing!" a friend exclaimed. Rachel adds, "Mommie told us when we grow up that she, Kathryn, and I should be a family band and hit the road, like the Judd family."

David laughs: "That's just like her—totally confident." Confident that she could excel at anything she set her mind to—singer, dancer, actress, tennis player, teacher, politician, mother.

"Why live life normally?" Martha often told the three, bursting with laughter.

Martha was our family's center of gravity. She was the communicator, the spark, our children's comforter and prompter, the puppy lover who kept things hopping around our home. I remember well the days she rushed Rachel to dance, Kathryn to tennis, and David to swim practice—all that after some city council meeting and before dinner and homework.

Doctor, Doctor

David sensed something was wrong a year before Martha's diagnosis. He was at Montreat for the summer. Martha was in the thick of her legislative campaign and flew up for a meeting. "She did come to our house to cook a meal," he says, "but she couldn't figure out where the pots and pans were. Grannymama had to show her. That really disturbed me. Mommie had no confidence."

Following Martha's failed campaign, Rachel came home from college several times during the fall of freshman year. She was upset about Martha's growing forgetfulness: "What is the deal? Why aren't you getting Mommie to a doctor?" I was as upset as Rachel, if not more. I'd been trying to figure out a way to get Martha to see a neurologist without further damaging her confidence, but I saw no opening. During that Christmas holiday, Rachel said, "If you don't want to talk to her, then I'd like to try." I finally set an appointment in the early summer of 1997. That's when Martha walked out of the doctor's office without seeing him.

Decision Made

"I can't think of a major decision in my life that she didn't initiate, even when she made me think it was my idea. She scripted my life, but mostly in a good way." When David finished the tenth grade, Martha and I agreed that he should repeat that year. His grades and behavior had slumped. Martha worked out a plan for him to attend junior and senior years in a different school system. *"Mommie was assertive but respectful through the whole process."*

Rachel was one of the younger children in her first grade, and that didn't work out well. Martha chose to discuss this with Rachel—what can I say?—in the middle of a creek in Montreat. They were hiking when Rachel was stung by a bee. They plopped down in the nearest creek, and while Martha put mud on the sting, she asked Rachel if she would like to be in her first-grade teacher's class again. *"Sure, I think so,"* Rachel said. Decision made, bee sting gone. This is typical of how Martha often worked—instinctively and off the cuff.

Blindsided

Thirteen summers later, Rachel had another important conversation with her mother in Montreat: "I felt like I'd earned the right to ask her what was going on, and I mustered up the guts to say, 'Any way you can go get checked out, Mommie? So we can know what we need to know?'" Martha said rather meekly, "Okayyy . . . it sounds like a good idea." Rachel let me know that Martha, having walked out on her first appointment, had finally agreed to see the doctor. I set another appointment and went with her for that one.

Receiving the dreaded news, Martha wanted no one else to know, including the children. I disagreed, but felt it was more important to let Martha have her way for now. We were dealing with enough confusion and fear. When Rachel called home and asked about the test results, Martha calmly responded, "Everything's fine." Rachel was relieved, until: "Later, in October, I was totally blindsided."

That October Martha finally agreed to let the children know the test results, but she insisted, "I don't want to be in the room when you tell them." David and Rachel came in, Martha hugged and kissed them, and then she excused herself. I pulled the door shut and turned to the children. "I need to tell you something; let's sit down. Mommie has been diagnosed with alzheimer's." I spoke in a voice more halting than I'm able to describe by writing. Rachel broke down crying, her body shaking. I held her, and David joined us in a long group hug.

I opened the bedroom door and invited Martha in. She looked at Rachel without saying a word, and Rachel looked at her. David describes the scene: "Mommie looked like a little girl, walking sheepishly back into the room. She knew she was in trouble because she hadn't been honest with Rachel on the phone a few weeks earlier. They collapsed in each other's arms, sobbing.

Rachel remembers: "I didn't really understand alzheimer's then. I just knew it wasn't good." And David: "The news of Mommie having alzheimer's was not a seismic shift for me. I didn't deny it, but I didn't sit with it too much."

Confident and Independent

Martha's confidence and independence breathes through our three children. David considers this one of her greatest gifts to them. Kathryn remembers playing cards in Montreat. "Mommie was so competitive. She didn't give me an inch as a child; she made me feel that she wasn't going easy on me.

"She was unafraid to stand up for what she thought was right, often pulling for the underdog." When Martha was a teenager she went to hear Dr. Martin Luther King Jr. speak in Montreat—in those days a bastion of southern Presbyterian conservatism—even though her grandmother told her she could not go.

Martha gave the kids permission to stay home from school if they were exhausted. She called these "mental health days." I first heard of these days when we were dating in Atlanta. She just smiled at me when I questioned her motive. David says: "Mommie was engaged with life and people, but on her own terms. She knew when to pull the rip cord."

Lost in Bitterness

Rachel spent her junior year of college abroad in Seville, Spain, followed by a summer internship in Jordan. She wasn't prepared for what has come to be known as *reverse culture shock*.

"I was a different person when I came home. I couldn't fit back into my previous role." Then at the start of her senior year, two years after learning of her mother's illness, a close friend from high school had a stroke, two best college friends had graduated, and her sister went to Panama as a volunteer at a children's hospital. "I no longer had a support network to lean on. Mommie had always been there, but now she was no help." Rachel cries as she recalls this period of her life. "Mommie and I always talked a lot, but talking with her on the phone now was almost impossible. I basically checked out of the home front. I was so bitter."

She recalls my saying, "You have to enter into Mommie's world now; you have to step into her reality." Once she understood that, she began to relate better to her mother. She began to see that Martha was incapable of responding to her in the way she had counted on.

I had my own adjustments to make. I had always deferred the role of family communicator to Martha. I now felt like a poor substitute—Martha was a real gabber and was attentive to all that was going on in the children's lives.

David recalls, as he says to me: "You had always sent my allowance check to school without a note. Then after Mommie's news broke, I started to get this epistle every three months or so, sharing what you were thinking." (That's when I began to send the children copies of my journal entries, along with a personal note.)

do-si-do

In her senior year of college, our daughter Kathryn participated in a poetry workshop with Natasha Trethewey, who later was named US Poet Laureate. Kathryn wrote nine poems themed around her mother's illness and its impact. She describes one of these poems: "My mother loved all kinds of dancing, but she especially liked to line dance with my father at the Joyland dance club. I start this poem in that setting to lighten the mood. It climaxes around my mother's first seizure. I was backpacking in Central America when I received the news. That was the lowest point in my life. I thought my mother was going to die. All I wanted was to go home—to see her, to hold her, to tell her I loved her. When I did get home, she and I went for a walk. My mother seemed to know I'd spent the previous twenty-four hours crying. By walking with me, she showed she wanted to comfort me, as I did her."

"do-si-do" by Kathryn Carlen Maddux

He remembers that night at the country line dance
club—Joyland on US 19—where he first saw her, and purposely
  knocked
over the Corona Light and pool stick at her side
(which he caught just in time) allowing her to say thank you with a hug
while the James Taylor hit from the jukebox became "theirs" from the
  moment it played.

He remembers her part in the already-scripted play
of their lives, as the instructor teaching him to dance,
him failing though, when he stepped on her toes and knocked
elbows as they tried to "do-si-do" side to side;
afterward all he wanted to do was thank her with a hug

but instead he had to work late at the office, not much time for hugs—
as she, alone, politicks it and choreographs a one-woman play.
Both out of sync twenty-five years later, the dance
comes to an end, her monologue interrupted, as sudden as the knock
of her head upon the ground as she lies fetal position on her side.

Curled up on the carpet at their bedside
shaking—and this time—giving herself a hug
he doesn't know what to do except press "play"
and "rewind" over and over again as his mind dances
and his body races for the phone which he knocks

onto the floor because now it's his knees that are knocking
but in his heart all along he just wanted to be by her side,
so he holds her head in his big gentle palms, wishing he could hug
her hard and upright as they did at the club, wishing he could be the
    playwright,
but instead is forced to watch the sirens dance.

It's Not a Given

Looking back over the years since Martha's diagnosis, David says the toughest part was spending a weekend a month taking care of her. "The idea of giving Daddy those weekends off was Rachel's. I was like, 'You know, that doesn't sound real great, but I guess I'll do it.' That forced me to face the issues and the feelings. Things like Mommie pointing at the mirror and yelling at herself, and then turning and directing her anger at me; that was the hard stuff. All of it was hard, I guess, but this was . . . more hard."

I didn't know Rachel had initiated the weekends, though it doesn't surprise me. I know they weren't easy for the children. These many years later I'm still thankful for those few days a month—they gave me time alone to sort through a lot of confusing issues. I wouldn't have been able to share this story without them.

David remembers: "A huge by-product of those weekends was getting to know Rachel again. Years of doing this caused us to rally around each other." All three agree that Martha's illness was a catalyst that helped our family pull together rather than drift apart. Rachel says: "We're now much more supportive of each other, probably more than we would have been. That's been a major factor in our getting through this. It's not a given that a family will pull together." Kathryn had a friend in high school whose mother also was diagnosed with alzheimer's: "When that happened, my friend's father left the family. She and her sister were forced to be their mother's primary caregivers and run the house while going to school. I can't imagine having to do that."

Yet those weekends weren't always hard for the children. Martha's sense of humor returned on occasion. David remembers lying on the bed with his mother when she got tickled over something: "I don't know when I've laughed like that." And then there was the greeting whenever David, Rachel, and Kathryn came into the house; I could only wish for such. Her eyes brightened as she rushed to hug them, babbling words that only she knew. Such moments of clarity and intimacy were a relief for everyone.

Greeting by Kathryn Carlen Maddux

Rachel peeks in from outside, Mom sits
on the oversized couch in hibiscus-pink
pants, a grapefruit-yellow blouse and rainbow-
striped sandals; Mom's typical outfit. She
is ready for the day, ready to have fun.
Rachel surprises her with a drop-in:
blinds bang against the wooden front door frame
signaling a toothy grin across Mom's face
and an echoing, songlike laugh as loud
as her outfit. Mom wants harmony added
to this melody, but she stops time. This is
the greatest moment ever—relived each
lunch break—made up of bear hugs Eskimo
kisses make-overs Patsy Cline hits, "Crazy."

David: Out of the Desert

   A year after Martha's diagnosis and just out of college, David followed his girlfriend and future wife, Katie, to Jackson Hole, Wyoming. "As a college athlete I had no room in my schedule for reflection." He was hoping to decompress as a ski bum. Instead, his feelings came unhinged. "I didn't have enough going on to cover up my desolation. I wasn't suicidal, but I did hit rock bottom emotionally. I wasn't in a great place. My trying to do my life hadn't gone well. I also was trying to figure out the God and Jesus thing."

David listened to the John Main tapes I'd given him and tried to meditate. He also read books by Frederick Buechner, Thomas Merton, and other spiritual writers. "I decided to try to let God do my life rather than me." On the beach while visiting Ventura, California, David stooped down, cupped up a big handful of the Pacific Ocean, and poured it on his head. "Baptizing myself," David says. "I didn't know if that was the right theology, but I really didn't care. Jackson Hole for me was the desert, and I was coming out."

Eighteen months later, David retreated to the Abbey of Gethsemani for a week. "I did a lot of meditating through the day, taking care of myself by letting God take care of me." David went to most of the daily Masses. In the evenings, he listened to the homilies delivered by Fr. Matthew Kelty, Martha's friend from a few years earlier. David was able to discuss with Fr. Matthew his mother's illness and its impact on us all. While there, David says he had no big breakthrough. It was more of a shift in which he allowed the issues in his life, particularly his work and his mother, to center on something bigger than himself.

Kathryn: Letting Go

A decade after her diagnosis, Martha almost died from pneumonia, and Kathryn spent several nights at the hospital watching over her mother. Upon returning home to Washington, DC, she sought out a therapist. The office was a converted house outside the city. A train track ran nearby. After a handful of talking sessions, the counselor suggested craniosacral therapy.

As Kathryn lay facedown on a table, the therapist applied light pressure across her back. Half-awake as a train passed by outside, her mind slipped into its rhythmic *clickety-clack, clickety-clack.* "That took me back to Montreat where I grew up loving trains. I saw Mommie and me sitting behind the Blue Cone, eating our ice cream dipped in chocolate, watching a train as it passed by." The memory of their putting pennies on the track came back vividly. "Mommie and I walked over and picked up the penny after the train ran over it." This precipitated a release within her: "I remember feeling Mommie was there in the therapist's room with me—just the two of us—telling me, 'Everything will be okay.' I finally was able to let Mommie go."

Rachel: Solace in Taizé

After graduating from college, Rachel planned a trip through Europe. Not long before her departure, Rev. Lacy Harwell came for dinner. As they talked, Rachel revealed the pessimism she felt about her possible career choices, plus the frustrations of being at home facing her mother's disability on a daily basis.

"Have you heard of Taizé?" Lacy asked. "When you get to Europe you might stop by there." Lacy explained that the Taizé

Community is an ecumenical monastery in France, which each year draws a hundred thousand young adults seeking silence and solace. That piqued Rachel's interest, so she and her friend included a weekend at Taizé in their travel plans.

On one of her first nights there, Rachel experienced "an out-of-body experience" in which she saw herself with her best friend from the University of North Carolina praying together in a chapel, something they had often done. She remembers: "I heard God's voice: 'Your prayers were not in vain.' As I reflected on this, it seemed like our prayers in Chapel Hill had dug trenches into the future, trenches through which those prayers flowed to protect us in our years of doubt and difficulty."

Rachel decided to stay for a week's silent retreat while her friend continued on. "I had the impression that I wasn't done with Taizé, and it wasn't done with me." Large gatherings and small meditation groups were scheduled throughout the day, but Rachel still had the opportunity to read, pray, and reflect alone.

"The main thing I realized out of this week of silence is that I felt abandoned by both Mommie and God. I was hurt more deeply than I thought. I hadn't understood how intertwined Mommie and my faith were. I cried a lot. I wrote in my journal, 'It's so weird for Mommie not to know what to do.' My crying was good because I'd been numb for so long." Rachel realized she didn't want to go back home and be around her mother day in and day out. "I didn't know how to love her without getting exhausted."

Rachel again heard God's voice, this time saying, "You will know when the time is right." She sought out a Taizé sister to talk about it. "I'd always had trouble making larger decisions regarding my life, and what I heard helped guide me. It still does." Rachel left Taizé with "a hope and peace that I hadn't felt in a long while."

Not the Final Definition of Life

Kathryn, when a college senior in 2004, said: "A painting of my mother's intrigues me.[2] In vivid blue, red, yellow, and orange, it shows primitive-looking ducks—a prehistoric kind that you might find on the walls of a cave—making their way past scrambled flowers and flying pitchers, toward a woman standing at her kitchen table peeling oranges. Reflecting on this painting, I saw my mother in a way that I had not been able to before. Although I had hints that she was more aware of her surroundings than she was able to express, I had not really grasped that. I'd been caught up by the 'fact' that she couldn't speak.

"My new insight emerged not only from this painting but also from the works of both a famous artist and a research scientist. The late Willem de Kooning was diagnosed with possible alzheimer's in the 1980s, after five decades of accomplished work. Critics dismissed his latter-year paintings as not of the same 'caliber' as the earlier ones. His use of vivid, primary colors supposedly wasn't 'serious enough' compared to his previous work in darker colors.

"However, Dr. Pia Kontos of the University of Toronto argues that regardless of any dementia, Mr. de Kooning's later work was as valid as his earlier. The conclusion she draws from her research cuts against the grain of our culture's mindless, and often crude,

---

2   This painting can be viewed at www.carlenmaddux.com/about/.

response to the mentally disabled. Dr. Kontos is convinced that despite any loss, such persons still retain an 'embodied selfhood,' and should be respected as such."

Rachel reflects on how long her mother lived with such a diminished quality of life: "I do believe that's where the mystery between Spirit and life comes into play. We can only see life as our reality of life—working, playing, talking, eating. But that's not the final definition of life."

Even in those later years, she sees that Martha's life had "tremendous value for her and others. Just in a different way than I would want."

A PASSAGE

We comfort with the comfort by which
we have been comforted.

—Canon Jim Glennon,
paraphrase of 2 Corinthians 1:4

Martha died on Monday, June 30, 2014, at 8:25 PM. That's sixteen years, nine months, and one week after she was diagnosed with alzheimer's. Six thousand and twenty-five days. She was sixty-six years old.

Neither I nor our children were in St. Petersburg. The four of us were in Montreat, all together for the first time with the children's families. "It was as though Mommie had wished us to be here when she passed," they said. The Saturday before Martha died, the last day I would see her alive, I told her that we were all going to be in Montreat. By all appearances she was incapable of understanding my words, yet somehow she knew.

When I received word from Menorah Manor that Martha was experiencing shortness of breath and a drop in body temperature, the first call we made was to Martha's good friend Jennie McCoun, asking her to check on Martha while I prepared to fly back to St. Pete. I was in Montreat for only one night.

"When I got to her room," Jennie said, "Martha was sitting up in bed looking out the window." Jennie kissed Martha while holding her left hand. "It was as though God were holding Martha's right hand," Jennie told me between tears. "This was a holy moment that's impossible for me to describe."

Jennie soon realized that Martha's breath and pulse were indiscernible, so she called the nurse. The nurse confirmed Martha's death and called me while I was en route with Kathryn to catch a plane.

I reached St. Petersburg on Tuesday. After wrapping up arrangements at the funeral home, I visited Martha's body. I was in a viewing room with Martha lying on the other side of a glass partition. The attendant permitted me to sit beside her, and then left. I held Martha's hand as I'd done so often at Menorah Manor. I detected little difference, other than that now her hand was colder.

As I reflected back on our lives, I slowly said aloud, between tears, our Lord's Prayer. This is the same prayer that years earlier in Sydney broke my heart apart, letting me see and feel my Father's heartfelt intimacy. And this is the prayer the children remember their Mommie singing in her pitch-perfect voice.

Sitting with Martha in this plain room, staring at two large furnaces, one of which would consume her silent and still body,

I heard Martha's voice singing this prayer. She sang to David, Rachel, Kathryn, and me—and to Christ Jesus, whose presence has been so real along this strangest of journeys. As her song came to a close, and her *Ahhh-men* led into perfect silence, I kissed Martha three times on her forehead, once for each of our children, and said good-bye for the last time, until we see each other next.

I stood up, walked through the door, and looked at Martha once more through the glass partition. I then walked outside into the fresh air, back onto the path that continues to unfold before me . . .

THE LAST PAGE

Dear Reader,

You've now read our story, or at least parts of it. And you might be asking, "So what do I do now? How does this apply to me?" My answer is, "I don't know; that's for you to figure out."

I don't mean to be a tease, though. As I look back over the years since Martha's diagnosis, I realize that I've talked with scores of people—spiritual directors, physicians, mentors, counselors, ministers, and friends—each on his or her own journey. Moreover, I've read dozens of health and spiritual books. From these conversations and readings—and from our experiences—I've learned some lessons that might be of value to you as you seek to discern the path you're on.

I want to respect our crisis—and yours—but one overarching lesson from our odyssey is this: "Lighten up." This type of journey, I've discovered, doesn't lead to ever-more depressing states of mind, regardless of the difficulty or circumstance. If the journey is authentic, it will make the load lighter. What did Jesus say?

"Take my yoke upon you, and learn from me. . . For my yoke is easy, and my burden is light" (Matt. 11:29–30). That's the guide I want to follow. And that's the trail I want to stay on as I move forward into the rest of my life.

Your crisis or story is not the same as mine, but we probably have more in common than we realize. And that could help us both. Some of my key takeaways are:

✓ Every crisis—be it health, financial, family, or relationship— carries a significant spiritual dimension. Learn to recognize it. It could save your life.

✓ This is a good place to remember that I dealt with certain spiritual issues through the lens of Christian concepts, vocabulary, and images that are my heritage. Yours may be a different faith tradition. Regardless, my story and yours should be about trying to survive. We need to be focused on figuring out what works and what doesn't, not on whether we have the "right" theology.

✓ Odds are that underneath every crisis is a serious dose of fear and resentment. Recognize these and learn to let them go. Psst . . . that may be harder to do than you think.

✓ Embrace your spiritual journey, but be aware that you could be forced outside your comfort zone. I was.

✓ One of the toughest lessons that I'm still learning is this: establish the practice daily of focusing on God, not on your angst-inducing problems.

✓ We're all busy. Yet no matter how busy I got during our crisis, I was forced to embrace intentional periods of silence. Otherwise, I would have gone nuts as my mind filled up with worries about Martha, our children, the magazine, finances, medical bills—you name it.

✓ Your path can be lonely at times, of necessity. But not always. So invite trusted guides and friends to trek along with you. And particularly invite those affected by your crisis, such as your spouse and children.

These are not all the lessons to emerge from our story; they're more like kick-starters. If you've stepped out on your own spiritual path, you probably understand what I had to learn the hard way: there are no shortcuts. If you'd like to join me in exploring these lessons further, please visit my website: www.CarlenMaddux.com. When there, you'll see a button to subscribe to my newsletter. Don't worry, it's free.

Thank you for spending this time with me. I hope you've found our story to be worthwhile.

[signature]

P.S. Several of Martha's paintings can be seen on my website, including the ones described in chapter 4 and in the postscript: http://www.carlenmaddux.com/about/.

P.P.S. *May I ask a favor of you?* If you've found our story to be meaningful, would you be willing to do two things? First, tell your friends about our book. And second, post a review of our book on Amazon.com. This would help broaden the reach of what many have told me is an important story to tell. To post a review on Amazon.com: (1) Go to the books section. (2) Enter my name as author of *A Path Revealed*. (3) Click the "customer reviews" link under the book title. (4) Click "Write a customer review." Thank you!

You may contact me via:

Website: www.carlenmaddux.com

Email: carlen@carlenmaddux.com

ACKNOWLEDGMENTS

"It takes a village," the expression goes. And getting the story of our family's odyssey to the public square has required that, and more. I started work on this book two decades ago, but I didn't know it then. From the time of Martha's diagnosis in 1997, I've slowly come to realize that our story is not ours alone, and that it had to be told. This story is for anyone staring into an abyss of unthinkable tragedy. My deep gratitude in this marathon-like effort is directed toward two camps—those who helped me bring this book into the light of day and those who, in one way or another, kept pointing us toward God's healing light during these years. Some family and friends bridge both camps.

First, I would like to thank our publishing friends. At the top of this list stands the entire staff at Paraclete Press. My editor is Phil Fox Rose. I've worked with a lot of good editors during my thirty-year journalistic career, and Phil ranks among the best. I quickly learned that he's firm, fair, and insightful. Equally skilled is the managing editor who works shoulder-to-shoulder with Phil—Robert J. Edmonson. They make a strong team. Paraclete's other staff members—marketing, sales, production, and distribution—are as professional as I've encountered. My book stands a much better chance of reaching its audience because of this able group.

Prior to Paraclete, I worked with an editor who helped me structure our story, Sarajane Woolf. By early training Sarajane was an architect, and that was a good thing because my manuscript required a lot of reconstructive work. Along with Sarajane is Carol Kline, a *New York Times* best-selling author who was my early memoir-writing coach. As I wrapped up my manuscript, Carol fortuitously reemerged and offered helpful insights on my book title and subtitle. I'm also grateful to Dan Blank, who's helped me develop my promotional efforts online, and to Robert Carter, who's worked with me locally to promote my book.

Next, I turn to those who have helped with the book's content. The feedback I received from a devoted band of early manuscript readers proved invaluable as I was piecing together our story. Half or so were longtime friends. The others didn't know us or the details of our family's story. Among the first I contacted were Art and Jan Ross, who read each chapter as I wrote it. Art is a minister, now retired, and Jan is an English professor with a sharp pencil and an even sharper eye. Invaluable as their insights were, the rekindling of a dormant friendship has proved even more so. In the foreword, Art's kind words help trace the arc of our story's meaning. He also introduced me to potential readers in Raleigh, North Carolina, and elsewhere—Laura and Steve Swayne, Zach

Clayton, Peggy and Bill Scheu, and Landy Anderton. I'm also grateful to another friend of Art, Rev. Dean Thompson, who insisted I work with a traditional publisher (like Paraclete) rather than publish the book myself.

Other readers who contributed in significant and intimate ways are Martha's girlhood friends from Montreat—Ellen Dean and Scottie Lindsay and their husbands, Dan and Scott, respectively. Also in this circle are Jennie McCoun, one of Martha's closest friends in St. Petersburg, and her husband Tom.

Rounding out my readers are those who played key roles in pointing us toward our path. The first is Sr. Elaine Prevallet, spiritual director for the retreat center of the Sisters of Loretto in Kentucky. Our friend and mentor Lacy Harwell told Martha and me in 1997 that he knew no one else with Sr. Elaine's gift of discernment. She is a rare gem. Second are Mary and Paul Zahl. Had Mary's path and ours not crossed three decades after our college years, this book likely would not have been written. Mary and Paul introduced me to their friend Canon Jim Glennon in Sydney, Australia. Paul, an Episcopal minister and author or coauthor of ten books, was most insistent when he said of my epilogue: "You need one more draft, Carlen; you need one more draft." He was right.

Friends and family lent far more than their moral support as we trekked along this path. First and foremost are our children, David, Rachel, and Kathryn, who also were three of my best readers. This path would have unfolded much differently without their heartfelt contributions. Next, our sister-in-law KK Cooper had an uncanny sense of how she might help. KK was the person who encouraged Martha to take up watercolor painting, and she helped us find our first caregivers. These caregivers truly made life bearable through the first decade of Martha's illness: Tricia DeRussy, Jancy Harvey, and Cindy Crockett. They quickly moved beyond their caregiving duties and became dear friends to Martha, our children, and me. When Martha moved into Menorah Manor in 2008, Beverly Wimberly and her staff made walking into that nursing home pure joy. Martha's family, of course, was there for backup support, especially her mother. Grace Elizabeth could be with Martha any time I had to be elsewhere.

There are too many friends to mention by name who took Martha to lunch, or walked with her, or picked her up for a church circle meeting. I do want to single out one group in particular, though—our Sunday school class. The core members of that class have for decades learned from each other and befriended one another. Perhaps unbeknownst to these class members (but probably not), they helped me solidify many of my thoughts, feelings, and impressions described in this book.

By now the reader should know that spiritual healing was an alien concept to me initially. And finding reliable sources locally proved to be difficult. But two persons emerged who were particularly helpful in suggesting sources: Jacklyn Williams and James Thurman, both out of the Christian Science tradition. Also, two ministers in our church contributed significant time and attention in the early years of our odyssey: Chuck Jones and Mike Davis. Through our mutual sharing, both helped me unpack a lot of feelings. And, yes, I would be more than remiss if I didn't express my gratitude to the brothers of St. Leo Abbey for their hospitality in honoring my privacy—and for making me crack up with laughter at their humor.

Meanwhile, as my focus was increasingly drawn toward Martha's care, many persons at our family's magazine helped keep it running until it closed in 2010. But two in particular were my anchors: Nancy Howe, our publisher, and Marcia Turner, our office manager.

Finally, I want to acknowledge some family members for their ongoing support, but who live afar. My brother, Bob, and his wife, Isabel, kept in close touch through the years. Thankfully, we had things to discuss other than issues related to alzheimer's. Both Bob and I have come to understand with a newfound appreciation the importance of family, especially since the passing of our parents and our sister. And our father's second wife, Lorraine, who in reality is our children's grandmother, has always kept a compassionate ear tuned to our needs and helped when she could.

Last but not least are two long-standing friends of Martha's and mine: Tom and Connie Elliott. We live in St. Petersburg and they live in San Francisco, so our times together in person, by phone, and by email have ebbed and flowed over the years. Tommy and I were roommates at Georgia Tech and at the University of North Carolina. And Martha and Connie shared an apartment at the University of North Carolina. Tommy and Martha dated in Atlanta. Tommy wound up marrying Connie, and I obviously married Martha. Weird, right? Over all these many years, I've never doubted that if I called and said, "We need your help," they would drop what they were doing and be on the next plane. That's friendship.

To all the above, and to those unmentioned, I offer you my deepest gratitude.

ALZHEIMER'S BY THE NUMBERS

Alzheimer's disease is bizarre. Over time, the victim doesn't seem to be in pain so much as the victim's loved ones. When Martha was diagnosed, a neurologist told us that a cocktail of medicines likely would be developed within fifteen to twenty years that would arrest the advance of this disease, if not reverse its effects. At the time of Martha's death, we were approaching year seventeen and research seemed no further along. Some statistics about Alzheimer's within the United States reveal the following:

- Alzheimer's is the most common form of dementia. Early symptoms often include depression, apathy, and difficulty remembering recent conversations, names, and events.

Later symptoms include impaired communication, disorientation, poor judgment, and difficulty speaking, swallowing, and walking.

- Alzheimer's is the sixth-leading cause of death and is the only one among the top ten causes of death that cannot be prevented, cured, or even slowed.

- Between 2000 and 2013, deaths attributed to Alzheimer's rose by 71 percent while deaths from other diseases declined during that time: HIV/AIDS, down 52 percent; strokes, down 23 percent; heart disease, down 14 percent; prostate cancer, down 11 percent; and breast cancer, down 2 percent.

- Of those persons with Alzheimer's, almost two-thirds are women.

- Those persons with Alzheimer's can be divided into the following:

   Under age 65—4 percent

   Ages 65 to 74—15 percent

   Ages 75 to 84—44 percent

   Age 85 and older—37 percent

- Of those persons 65 years and older, one in nine has Alzheimer's.

- An estimated 5.4 million individuals have Alzheimer's in 2016, which includes 5.2 million people age 65 and older and approximately 200,000 under age 65 with younger-onset (also known as early-onset) Alzheimer's. These numbers, though, tell only part of the story. For every person with Alzheimer's, another three or so are directly affected as caregivers, primary and secondary. And this doesn't include extended family members and friends.

- It is estimated that by 2025, the number of people age 65 and older with Alzheimer's will reach 7.1 million, barring any major medical breakthroughs. That's almost a 40 percent increase from 2016. A significant driver of this increase is the wave of aging baby boomers.

(Source: The Alzheimer's Association, "2016 Alzheimer's Disease Facts and Figures," http://alzheimerscareresourcecenter.com/2016-alzheimers-facts-and-figures-report/, accessed June 17, 2016.)

NOTES

PROLOGUE: A NIGHTMARE LAID BARE

Page xv *In a life of wholeness we may face brokenness . . . suffering is soul-destroying.*
Desmond Tutu and Mpho A. Tutu, *Made for Goodness: And Why This Makes All the Difference* (New York: HarperOne, 2010), 49.

TWO: TWO PROTESTANTS IN A CATHOLIC MOTHERHOUSE

Page 12 *You must stop examining spiritual truths like dry bones! . . . take in the life-giving marrow.*
Sadhu Sundar Singh, *Essential Writings* (Maryknoll, NY: Orbis Books, 2005), 101.

THREE: SMOKE SIGNALS FROM A MONASTERY

Page 28   *In meditation . . . we seek not to think about God, but to be
with God, to experience Him as the ground of our being.*
John Main, *Word into Silence* (New York: Paulist Press,
1981), 5.

FOUR: THE CLOSET

Page 43   *Don't deny the diagnosis. Try to defy the verdict.*
Norman Cousins, *Head First: The Biology of Hope* (New
York: E. P. Dutton: 1989), cover leaf.

Page 51   *Of the Seven Deadly Sins, anger is possibly the most fun. . . .
The skeleton at the feast is you.*
Frederick Buechner, *Wishful Thinking,* (rev. ed./ San
Francisco: HarperSanFrancisco, 1993), 2.

FIVE: ELVIS, DAD, JESUS, AND ME

Page 56   *Light breaks where no sun shines.*
Dylan Thomas, "Light Breaks Where No Sun Shines,"
in *Immortal Poems of the English Language*, ed. Oscar
Williams (New York: Pocket Books, 1952), 613.

EIGHT: A CREEK RUNS THROUGH IT

Page 101   *But we know, in some moments . . . fulfilled by eternity.*
Paul Tillich, *The Eternal Now* (New York: Charles
Scribner's Sons, 1963), 91.

NINE: MARTHA'S SONG

Page 116 *He who bends to himself a joy . . . in eternity's sunrise.*
William Blake, "Eternity," in *Immortal Poems of the English Language*, ed. Oscar Williams (New York: Pocket Books, 1952), 235.

EPILOGUE: REPORTING BACK

Page 122 Richard Rodriguez, *Darling: A Spiritual Autobiography* (New York: Viking, 2013), 3.

POSTSCRIPT: A MOM AND HER CHILDREN

Page 147–48 *Embodied selfhood.*
Pia C. Kontos, "The Painterly Hand: Embodied Consciousness and Alzheimer's Disease," *Journal of Aging Studies*: May 2003) 151–70.

CHRONOLOGY OF EVENTS

- **July 1996–July 1997.** The children and I detect signs that something is not right with Martha—occasional but notable forgetfulness, confusion, and depression. (*chapter 1*)
- **September 23, 1997.** Martha is diagnosed with alzheimer's. She turned fifty just twenty days earlier. I begin a journal that ultimately extends to fourteen volumes. (*chapter 1*)
- **October 1997.** Martha and I visit Sr. Elaine Prevallet at the retreat center of the Sisters of Loretto in Kentucky and meet Fr. Matthew Kelty at the Abbey of Gethsemani. We walk in the woods at Gethsemani. (*chapter 2*)
- **Late October 1997.** We tell our children about Martha's diagnosis. (*postscript*)
- **December 1997.** Martha and I begin the practice of Christian meditation. (*chapter 3*)
- **June 1998.** Our son, David, graduates from college, then spends the winter at Jackson Hole, Wyoming. (*postscript*)

- **January–May 1999.** Martha begins her watercolor painting class with our sister-in-law KK Cooper. Martha and I attend her thirtieth college reunion. We reacquaint with Mary Zahl, who subsequently introduces me to Canon Jim Glennon. Martha forgives her father. (*chapter 4*)

- **June 1999.** I begin an ongoing correspondence and telephone conversation with Canon Jim Glennon. (*chapters 4 and 7, and epilogue*)

- **October 1999.** I encounter Elvis, Dad, and Jesus in a reflection on a flashback memory. I forgive Dad. My love for him and God reawakens. (*chapter 5*)

- **May 2000.** Martha and I visit Mary and Paul Zahl in Birmingham, where he is minister of an Episcopal church. Their friend shares what I call a prayer-song with Martha. (*chapter 9*)

- **May 2000.** Our daughter Rachel graduates from college and spends the next year at home. (*postscript*)

- **June 2000.** I'm forced to take Martha's car keys away. (*chapter 3*)

- **Summer 2000.** Rachel and David begin to give me a weekend a month off, which I usually spend at St. Leo Abbey. (*chapter 3*)

- **July 2001.** I stay for a week in Thomas Merton's cabin at the Abbey of Gethsemani. I forgive Martha's parents. (*chapter 6*)

- **January–June 2002.** Rev. Lacy Harwell calls, and we begin a conversation that extends for six months. (*chapter 8*)

- **June–July 2002.** Martha suffers her first seizure. I visit Canon Jim Glennon in Sydney, Australia. (*chapter 7*)

- **May 2003.** Martha has a second seizure. (*chapter 7*)

- **March 2004.** Mentor and friend Rev. Lacy Harwell dies.
- **June 2005.** Mentor and friend Canon Jim Glennon dies.
- **January 2008.** Martha enters Menorah Manor nursing home. This marks the last entry in my journal.
- **February 2011.** Fr. Matthew Kelty dies.
- **June 30, 2014.** Martha dies. (*afterword*)

A SAMPLING OF MY READINGS
ALONG THE WAY

Spiritual Practice and Discipline

Athanasius of Alexandria. "The Life and Affairs of Our Holy Father
   Antony." In *Athanasius: The Life of Antony and the Letter to
   Marcellinus*, Translated by Robert C. Gregg. Classics of Western
   Spirituality. New York: Paulist Press, 1980.

Brother Lawrence. *The Practice of the Presence of God*. New Kensington,
   PA: Whitaker House, 1982.

Buechner, Frederick. *Telling Secrets: A Memoir*. San Francisco:
   HarperSanFrancisco, 1991.

Bunyan, John. *The Pilgrim's Progress*. Edited by Susan L. Rattiner. New
   York: Dover, 2003.

Cassian, John. *Conferences*. Translated by Colm Luibhéid. Classics of
   Western Spirituality New York: Paulist Press, 1985.

Chesterton, G. K. *Orthodoxy: The Romance of Faith*. New York: Image,
   1959.

The Cloud of Unknowing. Edited by James Walsh. Classics of Western
   Spirituality New York: Paulist Press, 1981.

Eddy, Mary Baker. *Science and Health with Key to the Scriptures*. 1890.
   Repr., Boston: First Church of Christ, Scientist, 1890.

————. *Prose Works.* Boston: First Church of Christ, Scientist, 1924.

Foster, Richard J. *Celebration of Discipline: The Path to Spiritual Growth.* Revised ed. New York: HarperCollins, 1988.

————. *Streams of Living Water: Essential Practices from the Six Great Traditions of Christian Faith.* San Francisco: HarperSanFrancisco, 1998.

Fox, Emmet. *The Ten Commandments: The Master Key to Life.* San Francisco: HarperSanFrancisco, 1993.

————. *The Sermon on the Mount.* San Francisco: Harper & Row, 1989.

Glennon, Jim. *How Can I Find Healing?* South Plainfield, NJ: Bridge Publishing, 1984.

————. *Your Healing Is Within You.* South Plainfield, NJ: Bridge Publishing, 1980.

Goldsmith, Joel S. *The Art of Meditation.* San Francisco: Harper & Row, 1990.

————. *The Thunder of Silence.* San Francisco: HarperSanFrancisco, 1993.

James, William. *The Varieties of Religious Experience: A Study in Human Nature.* New York: Collier, 1961.

Keating, Thomas. *Open Mind, Open Heart: The Contemplative Dimension of the Gospel.* New York: Continuum, 1997.

Kelsey, Morton T. *The Other Side of Silence: A Guide to Christian Meditation.* New York: Paulist Press, 1976.

Kelty, Matthew, OCSO. *The Call of Wild Geese: Monastic Homilies.* Edited by William O. Paulsell. Collegeville, MN: Cistercian Publications, 1996.

————. *Gethsemani Homilies.* Edited by William O. Paulsell. Quincy, IL: Franciscan Press, Quincy University, 2001.

————. *My Song Is of Mercy: Writings of Matthew Kelty, Monk of Gethsemani*. Edited by Michael Downey. Kansas City, MO: Sheed & Ward, 1994.

————. *Sermons in a Monastery: Chapter Talks*. Edited by William O. Paulsell. Collegeville, MN: Cistercian Publications, 1983.

Lamott, Anne. *Traveling Mercies: Some Thoughts on Faith*. New York: Anchor, 2000.

Lewis, C. S. *A Grief Observed*. San Francisco: HarperSanFrancisco, 1994.

MacNutt, Francis. *Healing*. Notre Dame, IN: Ave Maria Press, 1974.

Main, John, OSB. *Moment of Christ: The Path of Meditation*. London: Darton, Longman and Todd, 1984.

————. *Word into Silence*. New York: Paulist Press, 1981.

May, Gerald G. *Will and Spirit: A Contemplative Psychology*. San Francisco: Harper & Row, 1982.

Merton, Thomas. *The Asian Journal of Thomas Merton*. Edited by Naomi Burton, Brother Patrick Hart, and James Laughlin from original notebooks. New York: New Directions Books, 1975.

————. *Contemplative Prayer*. New York: Image, 1996.

————. *No Man Is an Island*. New York: Image Books, 1967.

————. *Opening the Bible*. Collegeville, MN: Liturgical Press, 1970.

————. *The Seven Storey Mountain: An Autobiography of Faith*. First Harvest edition. Orlando, FL: Harcourt Brace & Company, 1948.

————. *Spiritual Direction and Meditation*. Collegeville, MN: Liturgical Press, 1960.

————. *The Wisdom of the Desert*. New York: New Directions Books, 1960.

Metaxas, Eric. *Bonhoeffer: Pastor, Martyr, Prophet, Spy*. Nashville: Thomas Nelson, 2010.

The New Oxford Annotated Bible with the Apocrypha. Edited by Bruce M. Metzger and Herbert G. May. Revised Standard Version. Second edition of the New Testament. Expanded edition of the Apocrypha. New York: Oxford University Press, 1977.

Pennington, M. Basil, OCSO. *Centering Prayer: Renewing an Ancient Christian Prayer Form*. New York: Image, 1980.

————. *Lectio Divina: Renewing the Ancient Practice of Praying the Scriptures*. New York: Crossroad, 1998.

St. John of the Cross. *Ascent of Mount Carmel*. Translated and edited by E. Allison Peers. New York: Newman Press; Image, 1958.

————. *Dark Night of the Soul*. New York: Newman Press; Image, 1959.

St. Teresa of Avila. *Interior Castle*. Translated and edited by E. Allison Peers. New York: Image, 1961.

Sandford, John, and Paula Sanford. *The Transformation of the Inner Man*. Tulsa, OK: Victory House, 1982.

Sanford, Agnes Mary White. *The Healing Gifts of the Spirit*. Philadelphia: Lippincott, 1966.

————. *The Healing Light*. Rev. ed. New York: Ballantine, 1972.

————. *Sealed Orders*. Plainfield, NJ: Logos International, 1972.

Sellner, Edward C. *Wisdom of the Celtic Saints*. Notre Dame, IN: Ave Maria Press, 1993.

Sheen, Fulton J. *Life of Christ*. 2nd Image. New York: Image, 1977.

Singh, Sundar. *Wisdom of the Sadhu: Teachings of Sundar Singh*. Compiled and edited by Kim Comer. Farmington, PA: Plough Publishing House, The Bruderhof Foundation, 2000.

Waddell, Helen, trans. *The Desert Fathers*. New York: Vintage, 1998.

Yancey, Philip. *What's So Amazing About Grace?* Grand Rapids: Zondervan, 1997.

Health and Medical: Traditional and Alternative

Balch, James F., and Phyllis A. Balch. "Alzheimer's Disease." In *Prescripton for Nutritional Healing: A Practical A–Z Reference to Drug-Free Remedies Using Vitamins, Minerals, Herbs, and Food Supplements.* 2nd ed. New York: Avery, 1997.

Benson, Herbert, and William Proctor. *Beyond the Relaxation Response.* New York: Times Books, 1985.

Cannon, Walter B., *The Way of an Investigator: A Scientist's Experiences in Medical Research.* New York: W. W. Norton, 1984.

Cousins, Norman. *Anatomy of an Illness as Perceived by the Patient: Reflections on Healing and Regeneration.* New York: W. W. Norton, 1979.

————. *Head First: The Biology of Hope.* New York: E. P. Dutton, 1989.

Dossey, Larry. *Healing Words: The Power of Prayer and the Practice of Medicine.* San Francisco: HarperSanFrancisco, 1993.

Eisenberg, David, and Thomas Lee Wright. *Encounters with Qi: Exploring Chinese Medicine.* New York: W. W. Norton, 1995.

Gray-Davidson, Frena. *Alzheimer's Disease: Frequently Asked Questions.* Los Angeles: Lowell House, 1998.

Khalsa, Dharma Singh, and Cameron Stauth. *Brain Longevity: The Breakthrough Medical Program That Improves Your Mind and Memory.* New York: Warner Books, 1997.

Larson, David E. "Your Brain and Nervous System." In *Mayo Clinic Family Health Book: The Ultimate Illustrated Home Medical Reference.* 2nd ed. New York: William Morrow, 1996.

Mace, Nancy L., and Peter V. Rabins. *The 36-Hour Day: A Family Guide to Caring for Persons with Alzheimer's Disease, Related Dementing Illnesses, and Memory Loss Later in Life.* Baltimore: Johns Hopkins University Press, 1991.

Murray, Michael, and Joseph Pizzorno. "Alzheimer's Disease." In *Encyclopedia of Natural Medicine*. Rev. 2nd ed. Rocklin, CA: Prima Publishing, 1998.

Ornstein, Robert, and David Sobel. *The Healing Brain: Breakthrough Discoveries About How the Brain Keeps Us Healthy*. New York: Simon & Schuster, 1987.

Selye, Hans. *The Stress of Life*. New York: McGraw-Hill, 1978.

Simonton, O. Carl, Stephanie Matthews-Simonton, and James L. Creighton. *Getting Well Again: A Step-by-Step, Self-Help Guide to Overcoming Cancer for Patients and Their Families*. New York: Bantam, 1992.

ABOUT PARACLETE PRESS

Who We Are

Paraclete Press is a publisher of books, recordings, and DVDs on Christian spirituality. Our publishing represents a full expression of Christian belief and practice—from Catholic to Evangelical, from Protestant to Orthodox.

We are the publishing arm of the Community of Jesus, an ecumenical monastic community in the Benedictine tradition. As such, we are uniquely positioned in the marketplace without connection to a large corporation and with informal relationships to many branches and denominations of faith.

What We Are Doing

PARACLETE PRESS BOOKS | Paraclete publishes books that show the richness and depth of what it means to be Christian. Although Benedictine spirituality is at the heart of who we are and all that we do, we publish books that reflect the Christian experience across many cultures, time periods, and houses of worship. We publish books that nourish the vibrant life of the church and its people.

We have several different series, including the best-selling Paraclete Essentials and Paraclete Giants series of classic texts in contemporary English; Voices from the Monastery—men and women monastics writing about living a spiritual life today; our award-winning Paraclete Poetry series as well as the Mount Tabor Books on the arts; best-selling gift books for children on the occasions of baptism and first communion; and the Active Prayer Series that brings creativity and liveliness to any life of prayer.

MOUNT TABOR BOOKS | Paraclete's newest series, Mount Tabor Books, focuses on the arts and literature as well as liturgical worship and spirituality, and was created in conjunction with the Mount Tabor Ecumenical Centre for Art and Spirituality in Barga, Italy.

PARACLETE RECORDINGS | From Gregorian chant to contemporary American choral works, our recordings celebrate the best of sacred choral music composed through the centuries that create a space for heaven and earth to intersect. Paraclete Recordings is the record label representing the internationally acclaimed choir Gloriæ Dei Cantores, praised for their "rapt and fathomless spiritual intensity" by *American Record Guide*; the Gloriæ Dei Cantores Schola, specializing in the study and performance of Gregorian chant; and the other instrumental artists of the Gloriæ Dei Artes Foundation.

Paraclete Press is also privileged to be the exclusive North American distributor of the recordings of the Monastic Choir of St. Peter's Abbey in Solesmes, France, long considered to be a leading authority on Gregorian chant.

PARACLETE VIDEO | Our DVDs offer spiritual help, healing, and biblical guidance for a broad range of life issues including grief and loss, marriage, forgiveness, facing death, bullying, addictions, Alzheimer's, and spiritual formation.

Learn more about us at our website:
www.paracletepress.com or
phone us toll-free at 1.800.451.5006

SCAN
TO
READ
MORE

You May Also Be Interested In...

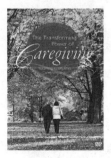

The Transforming Power of Caregiving

$59.95 Video
Running Time 48 minutes
ISBN 978-1-61261-6513

Whether you have cared for your loved one for one year or many, when it ends, it will feel abrupt. The life and routine that have become yours, suddenly comes to an end with a finality that is painful on many levels. However, exploring who you are, now, as well as what you learned about yourself – and about life itself – during your caregiving experience can be an experience full of discovery and adventure.

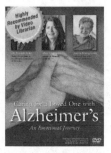

The Chants of Angels

$18.95 CD
Running Time 55 minutes
ISBN 978-1-55725-925-7

"Be transported to a place of timeless eternal beauty"–*Kansas City Star*

These ancient melodies of the church tell the stories of heavenly guardians, guides and friends, *The Chants of Angels* allows listeners to simply close their eyes, and be surrounded by these songs of prayer and comfort.

Caring for a Loved One with Alzheimer's

$39.95 Video
Running Time 50 minutes
ISBN 978-1-61261-240-9

This dynamic video offers insight, hope, and understanding for anyone who cares for a loved one with Alzheimer's.

Caring for a Loved One with Alzheimer's is divided into 12 segments and features lengthy interviews with these experts:

Mary Ellen Geist, former CBS Radio anchor, author of *Measure of the Heart: A Father's Alzheimer's, a Daughter's Return*

Dr. Kenneth Doka, Senior Consultant, Hospice Foundation of America

Joanne Koenig Coste, family therapist, author of *Learning to Speak Alzheimer's: A Groundbreaking Approach for Everyone Dealing with the Disease*

Available through Paraclete Press:
www.paracletepress.com; 1-800-451-5006.